Praise for "Goodbye Parkinson's, Hello life!

"This smart, soulful, and inspiring book will galvanize anyone who suffers from Parkinson's or wants to help someone else learn to live well with any kind of debilitating injury or disease. A fascinating hands-on explanation of how movement, music, and mindfulness can replace pills and pain."
  –Professor Susan Shapiro, New York Times bestselling coauthor, with Dr. Frederick Woolverton, of *Unhooked: How to Quit Anything*

"Alex Kerten and David Brinn understand the challenges of living with chronic illness and have offered a realistic solution. *Goodbye Parkinson's, Hello life* is clear, straightforward, and warm – a valuable companion for Parkinson's patients and caregivers alike."
  –Jessica Handler, author of *Braving the Fire: A Guide to Writing About Grief and Loss* and *Invisible Sisters, A Memoir*

"Each new person receiving a Parkinson's diagnosis should have the opportunity to learn they are still a healthy person... with Parkinson's. Alex Kerten's Gyro-Kinetics program vividly demonstrates that everyone – no exceptions – can choose to change their lives by taking the challenge to be a Parkinson's Warrior."
  –Lolly Champion, Education Chair/Vice President, Parkinson Association of Santa Barbara (PASB)

"His method also requires the mind to think positively: You are not a sick person who is ruled by Parkinson's, but a healthy person who just happens to have Parkinson's. The simple (yet challenging) shift in emphasis is a key part of the movement method. Kerten is refreshingly enthusiastic and encouraging, clearly explaining his method through very simple movement tasks outlined in the book. His method goes beyond being a dance manual though. It is a recipe for a different way of living with a chronic condition."
  –Dr. Sara Houston, principal lecturer, national teaching fellow, Department of Dance, University of Roehampton

"*Goodbye Parkinson's, Hello life!* fills a crucial gap in the emerging biotechnology advances. The power of what patients – and their loved ones – can do on their own is vastly underused in our consumer-oriented medical systems. I will gladly recommend this book to all our patients."
  –Jens R. Chapman, MD, Professor and Chair Emeritus, University of Washington, Complex Spine Surgery, Swedish Neuroscience Institute, Seattle, WA

"Alex's messages of living in attunement with our bodies, becoming more aware of the communication between mind and body, and the influence these have on our behavior encourage us to take responsibility for our own health, happiness, and hope."
  –Joanne Taormina, LMSW, Mindfulness-Based Stress Reduction (MBSR) teacher, Ithaca, NY

"Alex Kerten has created a proven method that gives Parkinson's patients hope for better coping and even improvement – using exercises and a new way of thinking. With the aging of the population, Parkinson's and other neurological conditions can strike virtually anyone, and his book will come to the rescue for many of them."
  –Judy Siegel-Itzkovich, health and science editor, *The Jerusalem Post*

"Alex Kerten's book proposes a proactive approach to Parkinson's – using body movement to combat nerve degenerative ailments. Movement-exercise systems are showing promise. May none of you need this. But get moving, anyway."
  –David Brin, bestselling author of *Existence* and many others

"This book is a statement of hope and possibility as it shows the limitations of our Western approach to disease and highlights the power of one's mind and perspective as it relates to healing the body. It's more than a regimen of exercises; it's a recipe for changing one's perspective and exercising mind over matter."
  –Lisa Wimberger, founder of the Neurosculpting® Institute and author of *New Beliefs, New Brain* and *Neurosculpting: A Whole-Brain Approach to Heal Trauma, Rewrite Limiting Beliefs, and Find Wholeness*

"Alex Kerten has given an answer to Parkinson's conditions for which there are no answers in any other kind of treatment. He strengthens not only patients' motor skills but also their confidence in themselves. I would recommend anyone with signs of Parkinson's to try Alex's methods."
 —Dr. Zeev Nitzan, neurologist, Barzilai Medical Center, Ashkelon, Israel

"The unique combination of music, dance movements, specialized massage techniques, and awareness of behavior works not only for Parkinson's sufferers but also for a large array of musculoskeletal disorders and other ailments. If your body is able to move, in addition to medication (when appropriate), it only requires self-commitment, belief in the ability of the brain and body to change, and it works! Results speak for themselves."
 —Pessy Benjaminy, Gyro-Kinetics practitioner, Spring Therapy Clinic, Edmonton, AB, Canada

"The body is life, and Alex shows that keeping the body graceful and moving through a challenge like Parkinson's is not only possible, it's something anyone can do. Step-by-step guidance is given for practical ways to deepen a connection to the body even in the midst of change and challenge. Through deceptively simple exercises, he helps readers to rewire their brains to increase their balance, strength, self-confidence, and most of all, joy at the miracle of life. This book is an integration of mind and body, movement and rest. It focuses on the whole person, from their mindset to their bodies to their relationship with caregivers. It shows that Parkinson's can be an invitation to reclaim life fully on one's own terms."
 —Keith Martin-Smith, author of the award-winning *A Heart Blown Open*, Shaolin Kung Fu lineage holder and teacher, and ordained Zen priest

"Alex Kerten is an expert guide at our side. Parkinson's sufferers particularly fall victim to adopting false and damaging scripts that must be forcefully discarded and be replaced with a life-enhancing one insisting on living in the present. We have to be aware and fine-tuned to the body's rhythms and desire to feel good. Alex's book is a great gift to all of us; may we follow its wisdom."
 —Harvey Scher, consultant, Weizmann Institute of Science

"How wonderful, encouraging, and spirit-nurturing it would have been to have a book like Alex Kerten's *Goodbye Parkinson's, Hello life!* Alex's holistic approach to body/mind therapy would have given my father the tools to overcome the ravages of his symptoms and fight Parkinson's as a warrior."
 —Arthur G. Insana, President/Creative Director, InsanaMedia.com

"Alex Kerten is giving sufferers of Parkinson's disease a way to fight back. Through a combination of breathing exercises, positive thinking, and music and dance therapy, Kerten has developed a strategy that he says can halt and even reverse the effects of this debilitating condition. In a world where more medicine is often the only answer, Kerten says there is another way, and he has hundreds of satisfied patients to prove it."
 —Josef Federman, The Associated Press

"You now have a choice. Yes, medication is necessary and important, but now you can physically do something to reclaim a pleasant and enjoyable life. If you are willing to invest twenty to thirty minutes a day to fight back, then read and initiate the battle plan contained in these pages."
 —Forris Day Jr., reviewer at ScaredStiffReviews.com, "Coffee Shop Conversations" podcast host

"Alex Kerten and David Brinn have written a sensitive and insightful guide that offers a real avenue of hope for Parkinson's patients and their families. Not only through its unique outlook on movement and rhythm but also through its plain talk life lessons, *Goodbye Parkinson's, Hello life!* should provide all the tools required to get you back on your feet both physically and spiritually."
 —Rabbi Shmuley Boteach, international bestselling author of 30 books and founder of The World Values Network

Goodbye Parkinson's, Hello life!

The Gyro-Kinetic Method for Eliminating Symptoms and Reclaiming Your Good Health

By Alex Kerten

with David Brinn

DIVINE
ARTS

Published by DIVINE ARTS
DivineArtsMedia.com

An imprint of Michael Wiese Productions
12400 Ventura Blvd. #1111
Studio City, CA 91604
(818) 379-8799, (818) 986-3408 (FAX)

Cover design: Johnny Ink. johnnyink.com
Book Layout: William Morosi
Copyediting: Gary Sunshine
Printed by McNaughton & Gunn, Inc., Saline, Michigan

Text set in 11-point Avenir Next with headings in 18-point Avenir Next Italic.

Cover photo by Debbie Zimelman
All photographs by Debbie Zimelman, unless otherwise stated
www.debzim.com

DISCLAIMER
Any information given in this book is not intended to be taken as a replacement for medical advice. Readers should consult with a qualified medical practitioner to determine that they meet physical requirements before undertaking any exercises detailed in this book. If exercises cause prolonged pain or discomfort, consult with a qualified medical practitioner immediately.

Library of Congress Cataloging-in-Publication Data

Kerten, Alex, 1945-
 Goodbye Parkinson's, Hello life! : the gyro-kinetic method for eliminating symptoms and reclaiming your good health / by Alex Kerten with David Brinn.
    pages cm
 Includes bibliographical references.
 ISBN 978-1-61125-044-2
 1. Parkinson's disease--Patients--Rehabilitation. 2. Conduct of life. 3. Self-care, Health. I. Brinn, David, 1958- II. Title.
 RC382.K47 2016
 616.8'33--dc23
                                    2015012172

Printed on Recycled Stock

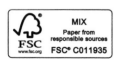

Contents

SECTION 1: GETTING READY

SECTION 2: THE EXERCISES

SECTION 3: KEEP GOING!

SECTION 4: ADDITIONAL READING

Dedication

by Alex Kerten

I would like to dedicate this book to all those who know the difference between being a "patient" and being a "client."

A patient will look for health with the help of God, an instructor, an MD, and with medication. The client will take what is needed of that help and understand that the phrase "with the help I give myself" is something completely different. The client is responsible for his/her well-being, and all the rest are means to achieve that goal.

Parkinson's disease has attached its behavior patterns to your body and mind. I hope that you will learn with time how to detach these unwanted behavior patterns and attach yourselves to new neural patterns that will decrease your percentage of Parkinson's, and introduce new habits of behavior that make you feel good.

Learn how to detach from your thoughts, change your body forms, expressions, and body rhythms and attach yourselves to a more positive, happier, and healthier act.

You can do it!

I wish you success.

Foreword

by Dr. Marieta Anca–Herschkovitsch

I met Alex Kerten because of my patients.

I was working with Parkinson's patients as part of a fellowship I was granted on Parkinson's and

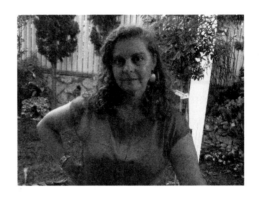

Movement at Ichilov Hospital in Tel Aviv in 2000 under the guidance of Dr. Nir Giladi, a world-renowned authority in the field of movement disorders.

Some of my patients told me that they were also attending sessions at something called the Gyro-Kinetics clinic, which was founded and run by Alex. I had no idea what they were talking about.

At that time, many in the medical establishment considered physiotherapy or any other kind of movement treatment to be the work of charlatans at worst, or placebos at best. There was little belief that therapy involving movement could be helpful.

But, as more and more patients explained to me that the Gyro-Kinetics treatment was changing how they felt, and as I saw this improvement with my own eyes, I decided to go see for myself what they were talking about.

I made an appointment and went to Gyro-Kinetics, met and spoke with Alex, and asked him if I could observe what he does. I watched his sessions with his clients and saw his integration of movement, music, and the physiology of behavior.

I was very impressed and immediately and intuitively realized that it was the correct approach and a fantastic development for Parkinson's sufferers.

It's been proven scientifically that movement and music open up new pathways in the neural networks, lubricates them, and enables them to work more efficiently. Alex, one of the pioneers in this field, took that concept and created something strikingly original and tremendously effective.

I suggested to him that we conduct a pilot program to check that effectiveness. We took 12 new clients of his and conducted a general overview of their physical and psychological condition. They then began Alex's program for three months and underwent another checkup.

In a subjective manner based on outward appearance, there was unanimous improvement in the subjects' condition. But also objectively, in the scientific scales that I conducted both for their physical and psychological state, there was also significant improvement.

In my conclusions, I wrote, "Gyro-Kinetics appears to be effective on general motor and mood dysfunction in PD. It can also improve respiratory and gastrointestinal disturbances and the patient's disease awareness. The combined modalities of GK provide a higher effectiveness and usefulness in the early stages of the disease in order to prevent the later complications."

In addition, another discovery was the decrease in the patients' dependence on medication.

For many of the cases, doing the physical activity for an hour provided the same results as taking the medication.

They entered an "on" position (a period when symptoms are somewhat under control) – because there's an immediate effect – and held on to it. They were able to skip a dosage that day, which is quite significant. Parkinson's sufferers can become obsessive with their medication, just waiting until the next time they can take it. And here in a deliberate fashion, they were saying, "I don't need it." This was a huge eye-opener.

Alex's uniqueness is the way he's helped his clients change their way of thinking about the disease. From meeting countless people suffering from Parkinson's, Alex came to realize that it was not simply an issue of problems with movement.

Movement doesn't work by itself; it works in conjunction with the brain. A person's psychology, mood, thoughts, and level of anxiety have a huge influence on his condition.

Therefore, Alex understood that the moment you can have an influence on the mind, it in turn can influence how the body behaves, enabling them to cooperate with each other. He understood that there's a connection between what we think, what we feel, and how our body behaves.

Awareness is a very important thing. In modern medicine, we tend to ignore it or have forgotten it. We take one X-ray after another and one test after another, and the human being is forgotten somewhere in the middle.

We take care of problems in the body – in the hand or in the leg – but we don't look at the entire picture. Because Alex does provide that vital integration of mind and body, and relates to each person as an individual, it helps the client to realize that his sickness is not the "end of the world" but like Alex says, he is a "healthy person with Parkinson's."

You can be a healthy person missing one leg, or a healthy person with diabetes. You can be a healthy person with Parkinson's! It's a very, very important concept that I learned from Alex, and I tell it to my patients all the time.

Over the last 10 years, there hasn't been a conference organized on movement disorders that wasn't full of sessions on music and movement, physiotherapy, the integration of movement and rhythm. There's blanket agreement that you can no longer treat Parkinson's — and all neurological diseases — with just medication and without movement.

I believe in the work that Alex is doing, and in his approach to his clients as healthy people with Parkinson's.

His treatment is not inexpensive, yet people make an effort to come to him from around Israel and from around the world. It's not easy for most of them to get there. It must be worth it to them. Because it works and because it makes them feel better. That's the quality assurance factor — if it wasn't so beneficial, people wouldn't be making the effort to come from all over to get his treatment.

Since I've known him, many alternative methods have been developed to treat Parkinson's using movement, but nobody has succeeded like he has.

Dr. Herschkovitsch is a neurologist, and the head of Movement Disorder Clinic at the Edith Wolfson Medical Center, Holon, Israel.

The Arts of Healing Movements: Alex's Story

My life has been framed by the shadows of two cataclysmic events: the Holocaust and the subsequent creation in 1948 of the State of Israel.

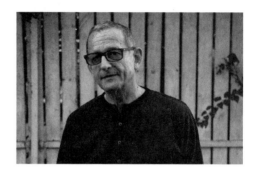

My parents arrived in what was then called Palestine at the tail end of World War II, both having made their way to that refuge from their decimated European homes. They found each other among the streams of immigrants pouring in after the war, and I was born in 1945.

The country was filled with fractured souls who had suffered the horrors of Nazi atrocities and been left plagued by trauma from the past. For many of the children of these survivors like myself, that trauma was passed on and became part of our own psychological makeup.

As a teenager, I discovered music as an outlet to lighten the heaviness that I felt as a child and the recurring dreams and nightmares I kept having about the Holocaust.

I threw myself into my new passion and, by the age of 16, I was playing the guitar in a house band that appeared on the radio, performed with leading Israeli artists, and accompanied visiting artists to Israel like Harry Belafonte and Jacques Brel. At 18, like every Israeli teenager, I was inducted into the Israel Defense Forces where I was first exposed to – and attracted by – martial arts (MA). After completing my mandatory service, I decided to pursue the study of martial arts in Japan and, later, when I returned to Israel, I continued the regimen under Grand Master Gad Skornic. After years of study, in which I also gained valuable real-life experiences, I graduated with seven black belts – four in *KenpoJitsu*, one in Ninjitsu, and two in Hashita.

Over the following decades, while pursuing various business pursuits, I continued to focus on the connection between mind and body. I began to study structuring and healing movements at the Dr. Aryeh Kalev Center, where I worked and taught the arts of healing movements for about five years. At the same time I studied psychophysical integration (or mind/body integration) at the Trager Institute, an approach developed by Dr. Milton Trager.

All of this research was spurred on by an incident that happened to me about 30 years ago during a martial arts training session.

I was choked by one of the instructors. He wouldn't let go of his grip. My hand paralyzed, I attempted to get him to stop by looking at him in the eyes. Instead, he interpreted the stare as a challenge and continued the choke hold.

All of my old Holocaust nightmares of torture and humiliation suffered at the hands of Nazis rushed back to me – and I fainted. That traumatic incident haunted me and developed into chronic dreams and nightmares that affected my life for many years. I looked for help by going to various specialists in the medical field, but nobody provided a remedy. So I decided that I was going to have to help myself.

I began to investigate the physiology of behavior – how our brain waves and the autonomic nervous system (ANS) in our body affect our anatomy, and how we live our traumas over and over again by entering into an anxiety-filled state of being. I began to realize that I was constantly repeating those horror stories about the Holocaust in my mind, and they were having a debilitating effect on my very being.

Building on my accumulated knowledge of martial arts and behavior patterns of the body and mind, I began to communicate with my body, instead of listening to the stories from the past being constantly generated by my mind; I managed to rid myself of my chronic nightmares and anxiety through mind/body interaction!

With time, I began to specialize in behavior patterns, body forms, art of movement, body language, the power of music upon our neural networks, and the effects they have upon our body systems. I honed the method while working for two years at the Reuth Hospital, and, later, at the Maccabi Health Institute, part of the Maccabi health care services in Israel.

It was then that I decided that I could share what I had learned with others who suffered from chronic disorders.

Clients came to me with behavior problems and unclear chronic diseases for which MDs had no answers. I built a methodic program in physical behavior patterns in which the clients learned about body language, mind language, and mind/body interaction while acquiring techniques to deal with their chronic problems.

I became skilled in various forms of physical therapy for pain, movement, posture, respiratory, and attention disorders. My specialty is working with Parkinson's disease (PD) patients, who, in actuality, suffer from a combination of the above neuropathological disorders.

Based on my knowledge in these fields, I developed the Gyro-Kinetic method, which is founded on the concept of movement, music, and rhythm – creating motion in the body, which stimulates simultaneous physiological, biological, and psychological reactions.

The unique combination of martial arts, movement arts, and the use of music is the distinguishing mark of the G-K method and reflects the multidisciplinary experience I've acquired during my years of training.

Instead of listening to their minds, I have taught my clients how to listen to their bodies and communicate between the two. Our minds are constantly dredging up stories and scripts from our past that dictate how we should behave, and we've stopped listening to our bodies. This simple but incredibly powerful concept is the key to my method and it has consistently proved its potential upon the symptoms we call "Parkinson's" and other neurological conditions.

I believe that what I teach and continue to teach myself in the fields of the physiology of behavior, martial arts, and the art of movement has a valuable lesson for everyone – especially for people diagnosed with early-stage Parkinson's. So join me as I show you how to retake control of your body, your mind, and your life.

Snapshot of a Session –
New Hope with Gyro-Kinetics

Entering Alex Kerten's Gyro-Kinetics clinic in Herzliya, a leafy suburb north of Tel Aviv, one is met with the soothing recorded sounds of a rhythmic orchestra. Participants arriving for the early-morning session straggle in – some on their own, and a few escorted by family members or caretakers. They all have advanced-stage Parkinson's.

Most of them tremble or have difficulty moving some or all of their limbs. But shoes come off, big blow-up bouncy exercise balls come out, and soon they are walking in a big circle – rolling and bouncing the round cylinders to each other.

One man in his 60s shouts out a thunderous "Hah!" every time he propels the ball off on a trajectory – releasing a deep breath from his abdomen.

Alex enters the studio, takes his shoes off, and crosses the gym mats to his DJ booth in the corner where he adjusts a head microphone. With a spry "good morning," he quickly changes the music into a rhythmic, upbeat disco tune.

The participants leave the balls alone and pick up the pace, circling the room accompanied by Alex's staccato instructions: "Legs!" "Forward!" "Breathe!" "Add your arms!" "Pay attention to your body, your breathing, your rhythm!"

Those who are able follow his lead, those who can't keep up the pace hold hands with each other and move their bodies the best they can. After five minutes, Alex abruptly shuts off the music.

"Pay attention to your own rhythm now – watch your body – ask yourself: How do I look? Am I stooped? Am I straight?"

The participants catch their breath while Alex puts on the ethereal, mellow sounds of Ralph McTell's "Streets of London" and issues new instructions: "Bend at the waist, feel the movement in your body.

"Feel it in your shoulders, ignite them, let your head move. Feel it getting looser. Little by little bend more, feel your spine, introduce movement and open it. Push with your fanny."

The more limber participants are back in the circle for the next phase, a marching song – upbeat and triumphant. "Find the spring in your feet – jump! Jump!" calls out Alex.

The participants jump and jump, to varying degrees. Some just continue to move however they can. When Alex puts on Elton John's "Your Song," and tells them to "conduct the orchestra," they each enter their own world, flailing their arms, tossing their heads and shoulders, and twirling around their legs.

The transformation for some of them, from the time they entered 20 minutes before to now, has been monumental. Stooped, brittle, and restricted in movement, they've become free-form dancers.

Lights out! Everyone lies down on the mats with pillows, legs extended as Alex puts on dreamy world music.

"Breathe in — your legs and arms are glued to the floor. Feel how the blood flows through your limbs. Pay attention to your spine and vertebrae. Go for a walk inside your own body, a sailboat through your nervous system.

"You feel connected to your body and all of your organs. They work together like a big machine in a factory — full of synergy and they are ignited by your breathing and your rhythm."

The participants slowly rise from their prone positions, the blood coursing through their veins with their diaphragms and abdomens synchronized in rhythmic breathing. An hour has gone by, but for them, it's been a lifetime. They leave the session to continue their day with the knowledge that there is a way to push aside their Parkinson's symptoms and move the way they used to. Their hope and their task is to make that hour stretch into a day, a week, a month, and a year.

— David Brinn

SECTION 1

GETTING READY

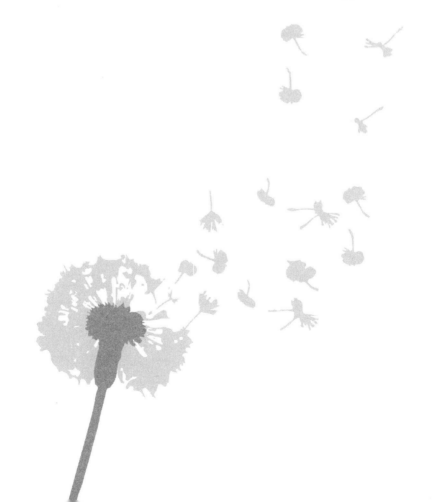

Chapter 1

Receiving the Script

You're probably reading this because you — or someone who is close to you — have experienced some of the symptoms of Parkinson's disease — the tremors, the freezing, the lack of control.

When you first went to a doctor and he examined you, he didn't give a chuckle and lightheartedly say, "Hey! Guess what? You've got Parkinson's, but there's no reason to worry."

Instead, he probably sat you down, and in a grim voice and with a sympathetic look, said, "I'm sorry to say that you have Parkinson's disease. This is a degenerative disease and your symptoms are going to get worse over time. Yes, we have medication that will slow the process down, but you should know that there are side effects involved."

That prognosis, quite rightfully, sounds like a death sentence — a movie script that ends in tragedy. What would be the natural reaction if someone received that kind of diagnosis? They'd go home, google *Parkinson's*, and get bombarded with ominous information and depressing photos and videos of Parkinson's sufferers and how they look and behave.

"THAT'S WHERE I'M GOING, THAT'S GOING TO HAPPEN TO ME!"

The script is now set in stone, and we, the actors, begin to play the role handed to us by the authority in the white coat. Our doctor has stamped our chart with Parkinson's – and he's stamped our soul with Parkinson's.

Without even noticing it, we begin to breathe less rhythmically, our facial expressions become more restrictive, our body language closes in or gets stuck, and before we know it, we've adopted the forms of Parkinson's. The result is that we've begun to act like a Parkinson's victim. Our performance is great – it could win us an Academy Award for the world's best actor with Parkinson's.

When Parkinson's symptoms rear their heads, we quickly lose our sense of self and our sense of confidence. We get stuck when we want to say something, we don't want to go out and meet people. We are afraid people are going to say, "Why are you looking at me like that?"

We're afraid that if we freeze, we'll hold up the line at the movie box office and we'll get razzed or snickered at. We are healthy people who have lost our movements and our rhythm. And we judge ourselves because of it.

Our behavior has become Parkinson's. It's marked on our body and fueled by scripts – stories generated in our mind that produce hormones in our body that cause us to behave even more like the Parkinson's victim that we are becoming. We live and breathe the behavior of fear, and we've acquired the chronic habits of Parkinson's.

It's time for us to say, "STOP!"

There's an alternative to the behavior of fear — it's the path of seeing the truth. We don't have to follow that script that compels us to enter the body forms and shapes of Parkinson's. Instead, we can learn to be Parkinson's warriors and break out of the harmful habits that have been slowly forming.

We can say, "No! I don't want that Parkinson's script anymore, I've been there and it's not for me."

That means we're going to learn how to feel good, we're going to learn about our body's rhythm and patterns, and pay attention to our body language and our facial expressions. By changing our script and eliminating our behavior of fear, we can bring ourselves back to a place where our natural movements dominate our Parkinson's movements.

We've unfortunately learned how to live with the forms of Parkinson's, but we also know how not to be in that position. We have lived without Parkinson's for much longer than we have lived with it. Even though it's much easier to behave like a sick patient than it is to behave like a healthy warrior, with dedication and the right attitude we can undo the chronic habitual behavior that our scripts and Parkinson's have thrust upon us.

We can bring ourselves to a new balance by becoming aware of our body language and the way it expresses itself with hormones through forms and feelings. We may put our faith in doctors or religion, but we also must take on the responsibility and put a little faith in ourselves. Doctors don't know better; we know better. But we don't always know that we have that ability. We aren't aware that we know how to "play" our body using the art of movement. Movement and body rhythms are the secret to feeling good and the basic element of life – movement is everything, for good or bad.

Once we know that, then we can change our relationship with our doctor – not as a desperate patient looking for a miracle cure, but as someone in control of the situation who needs some help. At that stage, the medication that doctors prescribe will be effective and beneficial.

We need to tell ourselves, "With *my own* help, I'm not going to be a slave to Parkinson's anymore."

Then something wonderful will happen. And we'll ask ourselves, "Where is the Parkinson's?"

Chapter 2

The Parkinson's Warrior

My gift is my ability to look at people and, based on their behavior, understand if they are balanced in mind and body. I examine their breathing, the forms of their abdomen and chest, the way their eyes look, the stories that their brain passes down to them from past experiences… and their future expectations of what Parkinson's is going to do to them.

Most of my clients are stuck inside these stories until there comes a certain point in our sessions when they realize something. The client looks at me differently, and I see a change in their body language, in their chest, abdomen, and eyes as it becomes clear to them.

"Wow, it is so obvious now. I brought Parkinson's upon myself."

One can develop PD through genetics or from being exposed to chemicals, but PD today is widely known to be a chronic disease brought on by our behavior. Therefore we first have to look into the chronic behavior patterns we've developed in order to begin diminishing the effects of PD on our bodies.

That's when we can go to work, and I can provide the tools to teach and guide the client out of their Parkinson's behavior. If we don't get to that place where we take responsibility for our own behavior, then it will always be a case of one step forward, one back – a constant zigzag. We must realize that medication, with its side effects, will not cure PD, but only delay it.

Parkinsonism

There are five stages of Parkinson's disease as defined by the medical establishment:

Stage 1: Parkinsonism

Parkinsonism means that you have Parkinson's but it's not professional Parkinson's. You have some symptoms but it doesn't have to develop or get worse and your condition doesn't have to deteriorate. At this stage, you can still change your Parkinson's script.

Stage 2

The symptoms are much more noticeable – stiffness, freezing, tremors, and trembling, a shift in gait, and changes in the facial expression are likely. There might be difficulty with balance and in retaining clear speech. The progress from Stage 1 to 2 can take months or even years – and if you've been able to change your script and learn how to communicate between the mind and body, it never has to get there.

Stages 3, 4, and 5

These stages of Parkinson's mark the major turning point in the progression of the disease. Daily tasks become more difficult, and your behavior patterns are unmistakably Parkinsonian.

Three Approaches to Parkinson's

I work with clients with all the stages of Parkinson's. But, regardless of their stage, there are three basic kinds of people who come to me.

- Those who say, "I have pain. Take the pain away."
I explain that I can take away the pain, but it will come back again and again. I help them to change their body language and their expressions – and the pain changes along with it. But they're unwilling or unable to change their Parkinson's script. So the pain and chronic habits will return.

- The second type of clients are those who are willing to work just hard enough to maintain their current state.
"I don't have the energy or the time to do this on my own, but I will come to you once or twice a week. You do your brainwashing on me, and I'll do the exercises," they say.

They are resigned to the idea that Parkinson's is always going to have the upper hand.

- The third type of clients are the Parkinson's warriors. They come to me to learn how to fight Parkinson's by taking responsibility through listening and speaking with their body. And they are ready to work every day on it at home, in between visits to me.

They are the ones who say, "I want to feel good."

That is such a basic and simple sentiment, but it's so important. If you're reading this, then you also want to feel good. And if you're a Parkinson's warrior, you can attain that goal.

MY DANCING WARRIOR

By SHMUEL MERHAV

Alex is my teacher, my guide, my coach, and my healer in my recovery journey. A year ago I was diagnosed with Parkinson's disease. It took me a few months to decide that I wasn't ready to accept the verdict that says that this is an incurable disease, and I became determined to find a way to recover. After a few months of searching, I found Alex. Thank God for that.

Alex is a dancing warrior. He is teaching me to become a dancing warrior too. He teaches me to fight. He does it by fighting alongside me and by showing me how to fight. It is not an easy thing to do, because Parkinson's is a very tough opponent and because I tend to give in from time to time and feel sorry for myself.

In these cases, Parkinson's wins and takes over my body. That's when Alex needs to fight me — my Parkinsonian side — until I refuse to give in anymore, until I join him and start to fight my Parkinson's with him.

This is a very tricky task: How do you deal with someone's despair and resignation and turn him into a fighter again and again?

By fighting me, Alex can easily make me feel like he is my enemy — which makes me want to refuse to cooperate. Alex needs to fight me in a way that will make me trust him, follow him, and join him.

So he dances. He dances with me, with my fears, frustrations, shortcomings, and despair. He listens to me. He understands my body and my limitations, and he leads me — as great leading partners do — to start dancing with him, and to start fighting my Parkinson's with him, not against him.

Then and only then — when he sees that I am ready — he puts on some great music and makes me dance. I begin to dance by myself while Alex instructs me how to move my stiff limbs and body and how to let the music guide them.

In every encounter with him I get to know myself and my body, my possibilities and limitations and the ways I can break my own limits. And I actually break them. My body, hands, and legs achieve a range of motion that I thought I would not get to anymore. My back is less stuck, my range of facial expressions increases, the joy and vitality are coming back to me and my body, and my walking is more energetic and light. As homework, I free dance every morning for half an hour and I feel much, much better.

When I first met with him, Alex did not promise to cure me of Parkinson's but opened a whole new way of relating to it, to my body and to the new situation.

In the first diagnostic meeting with Alex he said, "What I see in you, Shmulik, is 80% panic and anxiety and 20% Parkinson's. You are not breathing because of the panic. It causes your diaphragm to be stuck, and all the muscles in your back, shoulders, and arms adapt themselves to your locked diaphragm. We will begin to release your body from the panic and anxiety, and only then we will deal with the Parkinson's disease."

Alex explained to me that my anxiety did not result from Parkinson's disease, but an old anxiety that has been with me for years, to which the Parkinson's simply attaches itself. I understood well what he was talking about because I was aware of this anxiety, which has accompanied me for a long time. I told him, "If by working with you, I can succeed in freeing myself of this anxiety – I will thank God for Parkinson's."

And this is what is happening. Working with Alex has freed me from the panic and anxiety.

It is clear to me now that the Parkinson's is telling me: "If you do not start to live a full life, balanced, where your whole body participates, your Parkinson's disease will get worse. You will be stiffer, slower, shake more."

Parkinson's is the last call for me to live… to enjoy… to feel good in my body. Alex teaches me how to do it and I happily oblige.

I find that my body is now moving in ways that I thought were not possible anymore. And I realize that through the dances and the movements of daily behavior, I am succeeding in my fight against Parkinson's. I have begun to learn how to become a dancing warrior myself, just like my great teacher.

Shmuel Merhav is a management consultant and facilitator, working with CEOs and management teams.

Chapter 3

How to Use This Book

It's a new dawn, it's a new day, it's a new life for me…
And I'm feelin'… good.
— Nina Simone

The information presented in this book is based on years of research, work with hundreds of clients, and with my ongoing success with people afflicted with Parkinson's.

Used *in complement* with your medication program, it can show you the way to a much healthier life and state of mind.

You will learn how to feel good. And take it from me — nobody can argue with you when you feel good.

You will learn about certain behavior patterns that create chemical imbalances that take you away from your home-base center of balance and contentment. And you will learn how to regain that center by synchronizing your thoughts and your actions.

You will also learn that we are all actors, and life is a movie that we're acting every day. Part of our brain provides the script and another part directs the actor — the body — how to act according to that script. You will learn how to listen to what your body is telling you instead of what your brain is telling you. And you will learn how the mind, which has filled you with endless anxiety-filled scripts, can actually be the body's best friend and return it to a balanced state.

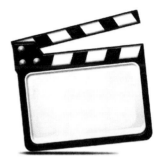

You'll learn how to be aware of the constant processing of these anxiety-filled scripts in your mind that lead us away from our home base. You'll understand how to stop them and how to be in the present — a state of mind that lowers your anxiety and can reduce your Parkinson's symptoms.

You will learn a series of exercises that will put you in touch with your body and the forms it takes and we'll explain the biological reasons behind those forms. Through focusing on breathing, movement, self-massage, conducting, and improvised dancing, you will learn how to regain your abilities that have been curtailed by Parkinson's — and with time these exercises will become part of your subconscious behavior patterns.

The art of movement, conducting, and changing your body language and facial expressions are all integral parts of an actor's repertoire. Taking on healthy body forms can in turn lead to a healthy body. If you can communicate health with your posture, your body language, and your facial expressions using the exercises in this book, it can lead you toward feeling healthy.

If you can't do an exercise at first, don't despair. The more you do and the more you include them in a regular schedule, the easier they will become. Using the information and basics provided here, you can build your own programs to enable you to customize according to your needs and capabilities.

Use this book as a guide that can be followed word by word and exercise by exercise – or take from it whatever you need to help you cope and overcome whatever difficulties you are facing on a particular day.

Parkinson's sufferers have good days and bad days, and sometimes you may want to concentrate on your breathing when you're trembling. Other days, you might want to focus on conducting and improvised dance to evict the forms of Parkinson's from your body.

Just remember, you can feel good again – and by working with me, you will learn how to become a Parkinson's warrior.

Chapter 4

What Is Parkinson's?

Parkinson's disease is caused by the progressive deterioration of nerve cells in an area of the brain called the *substantia nigra*. When functioning normally, this area is where chemical messengers called *neurotransmitters* are produced that enable our bodies to create smooth and balanced muscle movement.

When there's an imbalance of the neurotransmitters, it results in abnormal nerve functioning and a loss of ability to control certain body movements.

We can look at two polarities in our behavior – one polar extremity is survival syndrome marked by overstimulation, and the other is apathy, characterized by lack of stimulation.

People who develop Parkinson's have lost the sense of middle. It's been replaced by two polar extremes:

- dyskinesia: hyper, unintended, involuntary, and uncontrollable movements
- freezing: apathy and inability to move

Medicine and science have not discovered the reasons why the neurotransmitters become impaired. As we learned in Chapter Two, there are three primary reasons why most people get Parkinson's: genes and heredity, toxins and chemicals, and behavior

Behavior

The overwhelming majority of Parkinson's sufferers do not fall into either of the first two categories. The most common cause of Parkinson's disease is chronic behavior that affects and wears out our nervous system. This chronic behavior is the result of modern man constantly becoming entrenched in his survival syndrome, which affects the autonomic nervous system and thus directly affects our body systems.

If we accept this premise, we must then examine how modern society has inflicted upon us this chronic behavior of living in a survival syndrome.

What Is Survival Syndrome?

The root cause of most chronic physical problems today is our survival syndrome – a state of existence that we are all constantly living in whether we know it or not.

Before modern times, the survival syndrome actually enabled us to… SURVIVE!

Daily existence was fraught with danger. If we had to take a long trip through the wilderness, we'd be exposed to the elements; if it was freezing at night, we'd need to find shelter and hunt for food. Wild animals, seeing us as their food, were behind every rock as well as thieves who

would kill us for the
clothes on our backs.

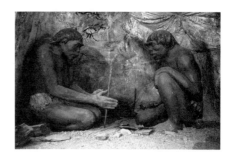

Our instincts and sense
of self-preservation
placed our ancestors
in a high-alert mode
as they coped with
the basics of survival – the three Fs – FIGHT, FREEZE,
or FLIGHT.

Today, unless we're on the front lines of battle, we rarely
face situations like that. In modern society, we no longer
need to kill for our food – we go to the supermarket. We're
no longer afraid of a wild animal killing us on a journey. We
take our gas-guzzling SUV. Life is easy, life is good.

Our survival syndrome is still there, of course. It kicks in
when we need adrenaline, when we're on a deadline
at work, when we're competing in a sporting event.
There are certainly times and places when we need our
survival syndrome.

The problem arises when our survival syndrome
becomes the NORM – and a chronic part of our lives.
When our home base is our survival syndrome, we are
headed for trouble.

In the modern world, our survival syndrome is triggered
by different stimuli than what moved our ancestors to
action: the media. We've become slaves of the media
and the stories they create.

We see "perfect" people on TV and in movies, we see what we can't have – whether it be the sports car, the beautiful model, or the white teeth. And we've learned how to be resentful and to feel inadequate, wracked with anxiety and self-doubt.

Without even knowing it, those thoughts have permeated our thinking, and our mind has been conditioned to work overtime, causing our survival syndrome to kick in.

Our survival syndrome brings us to fear – and that fear is actually what wears out our autonomic nervous system and alters our chemical balance.

Where Do Trauma and Anxiety Come From?

I've sat with hundreds of Parkinson's clients, and I analyze their lives, and observe their behavior and their spirit. And in most cases, I'm able to pinpoint the place it all began. Usually it's the result of a traumatic experience in their life, or a sense of constantly spinning the wheel in order to survive, not living life the way they want, a sense of not being respected by family or peers – or just plain anxiety.

Dream Scenarios

Have you had a traumatic dream that keeps on cropping up at intervals? Many of them are based on snippets of information we have internalized years ago, sometimes even as a child, and manifest themselves as behavior patterns that recur because of that experience.

Like I described in my foreword, many of us have recurring dreams of a traumatic experience from our lives that put us into a state of high anxiety, even while we sleep. We're filled with stress without even realizing it, until it becomes a chronic condition.

Everyone has his own trauma brought on by family and our reservoir of experiences, and they are alive and well in our subconscious. So without realizing it, by surrounding ourselves with these dream scripts, we've entered our survival syndrome filled with anger, fear, and abandonment – even in our sleep. We feel anxiety but we don't understand where it's coming from. So even if we think we're fine in our waking hours, we could be behaving in a high-anxiety level while we're asleep.

Chapter 5

Our Alpha and Beta States of Being

Two of the most important needs any person has are to feel love and support. And if we lack them, we feel abandoned and leave the door wide open for anxiety and fear to take over our minds and our lives.

Anxiety and fear are the chronic diseases of the world. We are not even aware that we have become chronic storytellers who trigger these harmful feelings.

The more stories that our brain devises, the less our body has control over what is happening to it. Because of our chronic mind behavior, the body is being dictated to as to how it should behave, leading us to enter our survival syndrome.

We live the story and we behave the story. Stories are ALIVE and they create our physical world. Most of the time, our scripts are based on our past experiences or our future expectations, and we're not even aware of the fact that we've left the PRESENT.

Our scripts are the stories we build in our neural network. They affect our *autonomic nervous system* (ANS) which in turn impacts greatly on our breathing, our heartbeat, our sight, our body language and forms, our digestion, our brain waves — everything!

Each script that we act out has an effect on our state of balance and our alpha and beta brain waves.

Alpha and Beta States

We mentioned feeling good. But what does it actually mean? The way we feel is determined by our brain waves.

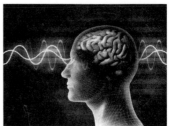

- ALPHA: We're in our home base of a balanced state — feeling creative, supported, and self-confident.

- BETA: We feel alert, hyperstimulated on the way toward our survival syndrome. It's when our "fight or flight" instincts and reactions kick in. It's also the state in which we feel abandonment. "I'm alone! I'm not good enough!"

As long as we can eventually return to our alpha state home base, the beta brain-wave state is necessary and beneficial to us. However, if we're in an artificial survival syndrome created by nonstop stories from the past and from the future, we are in danger of remaining in that constant state of survival, a situation that opens the floodgates to chronic behavior and conditions.

We don't need to talk about extreme life-or-death situations. It can be something as innocuous as the

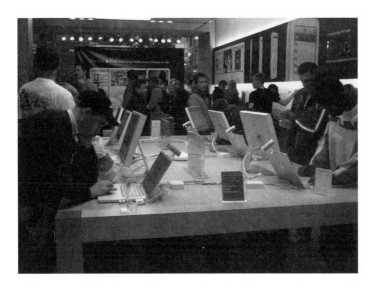

release of the latest smartphone. The media brainwashes us into thinking that we're not going to be able to survive, never mind keep up with the Joneses, unless we are first in line on Friday to purchase the latest communication device.

"If I don't get it, I'm going to miss out, everyone else will have it, my life will be incomplete!"

Instead of being in an alpha state, our new home base is now the beta state, and that's when the danger of psychological and physiological damage is rife. Without even paying attention, we've entered a permanent survival syndrome. And what happens to our physiology? We're wearing it out — burning ourselves out. That exposes us to any number of chronic health issues, ranging from migraines to chronic fatigue syndrome… to Parkinson's.

NEUROTRANSMITTERS

Neurotransmitters are the brain chemicals that communicate information inside our brain and to the rest of our body. The brain uses the neurotransmitters to execute our most important bodily functions – telling our heart to beat, our lungs to breathe, our stomach to digest, and other vital tasks.

When they're out of balance, they can affect virtually every aspect of our being – our mood, sleep, weight, and health. In addition to diet, genetic disposition, drugs, and alcohol, stress and anxiety can cause our neurotransmitters to veer out of balance.

There are two types of neurotransmitters: *inhibitory* ones (serotonin and GABA) that calm the brain and create balance and *excitatory* ones (dopamine and acetylcholine), that stimulate the brain. When the excitatory neurotransmitters are overactive, they can easily deplete the inhibitory ones to create a chemical imbalance.

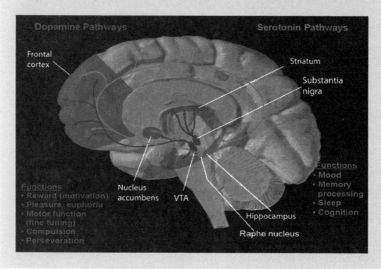

Chapter 6

Where Do Our Scripts Come From?

The Script and the Director

We are brainwashed all the time – but we are almost never "bodywashed." When we're growing up, do any of our role models – be it our parents, our teachers, or our religious leaders – ever give us this advice? "Listen to your body." No, instead we're constantly told: Use your brain.

Throughout our lives, we have been educated that we have a brain – our logic is in our left hemisphere and our emotions are in our right hemisphere. But we are never taught that we have a body that also thinks! Instead, we dutifully behave according to the way our brain instructs us.

The Script, the Director, and the Actor

Our brain's left hemisphere is the scriptwriter, bringing in information externally in full sentences – "I am starting a new job today, how will they accept me?" "My marriage is falling apart, what am I going to do?"

Our right hemisphere is the director – it reacts to feelings, body language, and forms by communicating through emotions and commands: happy, sad, hungry, tired. And it then directs the actor in this play – the body – how to act.

This process describes how most of us behave and I'm here to tell you that it DOES NOT WORK. It only demonstrates how we have lost contact with ourselves.

How is it supposed to work? In reality, our body is not just the actor in our play. Our body is much smarter than we give it credit for. We feel with our body, and we have instincts in our body via our autonomic nervous system, which affects all of our body's systems. Our body actually reacts much faster than our brain. The next time you put your finger on a hot stovetop, you'll know what I mean.

Just as an experienced actor can tell the director that the instructions he's getting for the scene aren't working for him, the body can politely tell the mind, "No thank you, I don't want this Parkinson's part. I've done it before, it's not good for me anymore. Stop! Enough! I want to change the story and take on a new role. I don't want to remain 'stuck' in the role of the past. I want a healthier role in the present."

Sentences Versus Words

Our nonstop scripts are communicated to the director through sentences: "I need to buy that dress right now." "I can't go to my son's game because this project is due in the morning." "I'm afraid to go to the restaurant because of my tremors."

When we speak with sentences, there can be judgments, disagreements, or arguments pitting sentence versus sentence. And it's enough to drive someone crazy – crazy with anxiety over the sentences zinging back and forth between the scriptwriter and the director... until it becomes chronic.

However, the director who receives these sentences communicates them to the actor – the body – in those more concise bursts of words and phrases: "Good." "Be careful." "Do it." "Stop."

The director is therefore in a position to fend off the anxiety brought upon the body. The word is more powerful than the sentence, and the timely and wise advice given by the director to the actor can help us change our scripts.

With one word, the body can change immediately. When the scripts are bombarding the director, all it really needs to transfer to the body are catchphrases like "Feel good," "Be aware," and "Don't think."

The actor can then change what is written in the script he was given. "I understand the situation and I don't want it, it doesn't suit me."

Once we get used to speaking in words instead of sentences, our life changes. Who controls the script? Our body.

Chapter 7

The Third Hemisphere: The Body

We've talked about the brain's left and right hemispheres, but we don't usually relate to what I call the "body hemisphere" because we're not really aware of it. Most of the time, we're constantly ping-ponging back and forth between the script and the director. There are all kinds of names that have been used to label this process – ego, self, subconscious.

But what's missing in the equation is what I call the third hemisphere – the body.

If the three parts of the equation don't speak together and work together, it will be like any government – total chaos. And that's what Parkinson's is – chaos.

Out of our three brains – the left hemisphere, the right hemisphere, and the body – the most important one is by far the body.

We might think we're doing everything to take care of our body – we walk on the treadmill, we play tennis, we meditate and do yoga. But still, something is wrong.

The Body Speaks

The problem is we're doing all of these activities through our head, not our body.

That's a major mistake, because the body tells us everything.

"You've been overdoing it."

"You're hurting me."

The body says everything and we ignore it. We listen to the brain instead and that's from where our problems derive.

It's the actor – our body – who says, "I know who I am, I know what I'm worth. I'm going to decide what the script is and what the director should do – because I'm in charge."

But, we've been trained not to listen to the body. Instead, we keep loading more and more scripts until we have activated our survival syndrome and worn the body down, making it susceptible to a chronic disease like Parkinson's.

We modern humans have stopped asking our body how it feels, and we're not telling our body "thank you." We don't ask, "Why are you so tired, why do you want to sleep all the time?"

Our body will tell us if we listen. This is what it might say:

"I'm tired because I'm running away. I'm fed up because I'm not being listened to. I feel sad – look how sad my eyes are, look at the form my body is taking – see how my chest is deflated, how my abdomen in constricted. See how sad I am? I'm sad because you're not listening to me.

"If you continue to behave this way and don't stop, I'm going to end up giving you a present as a wake-up call – Parkinson's disease."

A Client Encounter

FEELING THE PAIN

A client arrived in a wheelchair.

When I asked him the basic questions, he answered right away.

"I got Parkinson's because I burnt myself out in life."

I looked at his medication list and told him, "You are addicted to medication. You're living according to the clock and your next dosage. You have lost all contact with your body."

"It's so true, I didn't respect my body at all."

He agreed to fight like a Parkinson's warrior, and we started to work on the exercises.

"Close you eyes and pay attention to what's happening in your body. Feel your abdominal cavity, your chest cavity. What do you feel there?"

"So much pain," he said.

"Pay attention to that pain, feel it. Breathe the pain."

His chest began to inflate and deflate more noticeably.

"What do you feel now?"

"Pain."

"Is it the same pain?"

"No," he said. "It's different."

"Pay attention to that pain, breathe into it. Now tell me, why is that pain there?"

"It goes far back, so far back. I was never respected," he says. "I was always in a rush, I never took a chance to slow down."

"Now, open your eyes. How do you feel?"

"I feel pain still, but I feel better. I feel different."

He was breathing more easily, speaking more rhythmically, with fewer tremors.

"What I want you to do is stand up," I said. "Just stand. Sway yourself from side to side and continue breathing rhythmically."

He did.

"Now, lift one leg, and we're going to change the way you walk."

He started to move, saying, "I can't believe it."

"I want you now to go consult with your doctor so that step by step, you can decrease the amount of medication that you're taking."

After a couple more sessions, he arrived one day without a wheelchair.

"How do you feel?"

"I don't know, but I'm doing all kinds of things I couldn't do before. All I know is that when I went to the doctor feeling worse and worse, he gave more medication."

I told him, "That's because you've now learned that there are times when you can take less medication and instead take responsibility for your own well-being — and you feel better."

He had begun to talk with his body and by disciplining himself, was able to change his script. He was in a better relationship with his body and became aware of its demands.

He became a Parkinson's warrior.

Chapter 8

Physiology of Behavior

I'm a specialist in the physiology of behavior. I know how to look at a person and by observing the way he breathes, the way he sits, what he does with his hands, how he speaks, how he looks, and his body rhythms, I'm able to assess and understand what his problems are. That's because he is telling me what his story is through his body language.

The medical world looks at a person's psychology and biology, but they ignore his physiology. It's not yet in the vocabulary of conventional medicine.

Doctors have examined my work over the last 20 years and say, "We don't know how he does what he does."

Not long ago, a whole group of Parkinson's specialists from a major medical center in Israel came to my clinic. I explained what I do and related some of the successes I've had with my Parkinson's clients.

The head of the department turned to one of his colleagues and said, "Why can't we do what he does?" The answer the colleague gave was very revealing.

"We can't do it because we don't speak his language."

The physiology of behavior means that our behavior patterns are based on how our nervous system reacts to situations.

The physiology of behavior = behavior patterns = body language = movement and feelings within our muscles and nerves sparked by hormones.

Our biochemistry and our psychology start to change as we learn to control our way of thinking. They begin to interact through body/mind awareness and language, and when they do that, we begin to see a change in our physiology. And that's when we begin to feel good!

If our PHYSIOLOGY (our body behavior and feelings) and BIOLOGY work together, we'll discover that our PSYCHOLOGY will tell us exactly what it wants. I call it the PBP formula.

It's not going to be easy. We can always feel what is happening to our body. And it's not always good.

If we don't feel good, acknowledge it. Feel the feeling of not feeling good! Feel the forms of Parkinson's. Feel it within the abdomen, chest cavity, diaphragm, heart, and face. We will discover that we've adopted the forms of not feeling good.

That's a breakthrough! When we become aware of it, we can do something about it. The body can – and will – change because it is now focused on feeling good and striving to be healthy.

A Client Encounter

CHRONIC GUILT AND ANXIETY

I took on a client once. When she came for her initial visit, I looked at her body language — her abdomen was swollen, her chest deflated, her eyes sunken and sad.

"Why did you come to me?" I asked.

"I have Parkinson's," she said in a depressed voice. She didn't sing out in a happy tone — "Shooby dooby — I HAVE PARKINSON'S."

I asked her a question: "How much Parkinson's do you have?" She said, "I don't know." I said, "Maybe you have a little Parkinson's and a lot of anxiety.

"Did you experience anxiety before you had Parkinson's?" I asked.

"All my life was anxiety," she answered.

From continuing to talk to her, I gleaned that her behavior was based on something that started happening to her years ago. She felt chronic guilt and anxiety. Even when something good happened in her life, she continued to blame herself for her present condition and didn't allow herself to be happy. She turned everything positive into a negative.

When I told her about my observations, something happened to her. The expression on her face changed, she became more alert and wide-eyed. Her body opened up and changed its forms.

I was speaking to her body and it reacted. Her body said, "Wow, you're so right."

I asked her what kind of work she did, and she began to meander: "Well, I do some painting now, but I don't consider that a career. I had a serious job... but... I don't really know what I do now."

I said, "I'm going to stop you now and repeat what you said. 'Blah blah blah.' All your life you've been talking like this trying to explain yourself. But psychologically, you don't know. But your body does know.

"So now, let's try this again. Are you good at your work?"

"Yes, very good."

"Are you happy?"

"No."

"Who is not happy?"

"I'm not happy."

"Who is 'I'?"

She put her hands on her head.

"Now, tell me where do you feel you're not happy?"

She felt all over her body – "Here and here, and here."

"So why did you put your hands on your brain when I asked you who 'I' was? It's your body that's not happy."

She said, "Wow, I never thought about it that way."

I told her, "Your body is telling you 'I'm not happy.' Did you listen to your body? Did you ask your body, 'Is what I'm doing something that is good for my body or bad for my body?'"

She said, "Unbelievable."

I took her on the mats, where I led her in free dancing, conducting, and internal massage.

She forgot her Parkinson's story, changed her facial expressions, moved her hands, and exercised parts of her body that had been blocked. She was feeling good.

"When you feel bad," I told her, "put on music, close yourself off in a room, and do what I taught you. You have to learn to stop acting the script you were given, change the script by entering a different world with music, move your body and leave the forms of Parkinson's."

Chapter 9

Living in the Present

Free your mind and the rest will follow.
– En Vogue

The human brain lives the past, the present, and the future. And therein lies all of our problems.

With our developed brain, we have amazing ability. Our frontal lobes separate us from other mammals with their ability to incorporate the past, present, and future to analyze situations and conduct an internal dialogue. We send the conclusions of that dialogue to the limbic system in our temporal lobe.

The limbic system contains all of our knowledge and experience. Our mammalian brain lives in the past and the present only — as it stores and retrieves our memory and collective experience and instructs the body how to react. Our past stories and scripts are inscribed in our limbic system and have a major impact on our autonomic nervous system and, therefore, on our body.

Because our human brain can also plan for the future, it uses the accumulated knowledge and experience stored in the limbic system to create stories and scripts of how things might be.

But what if the script is fiction and isn't true? We are living a story that is not in the present, it's in the future and it may not even happen!

The result is that far too often, we are living in the future instead of the present, based on our past experiences. It's true for Parkinson's sufferers and it's true for all humans. We act out scripts from the future based on experiences from the past.

But by living the past and the future, we forget the present! We build stories and act those stories as if the future was the present. This constant thinking, analyzing, and script creation has a direct effect on our limbic system and our autonomic nervous system.

We think about Parkinson's and what will happen if we can't move our hands or get stuck in a public place, and we begin to behave the future until it becomes habitual.

But what if we can say, "NO, this script isn't accurate — I'm not there yet, I can stop it."?

The way we stop it is remaining in the present, understanding that we are not really in the survival mode that our script told us we were in. We've manifested the body language, breathing, and heartbeat from a negatively imagined future.

We can change these forms back to the present. And we can talk to our body and thank it.

"Thank you for the signs you are sending me about Parkinson's as a reminder of where I was headed. And thank you for telling me that I don't have to continue going there."

Chapter 10

Regaining the Middle

Once we're aware that our scripts have been burning out our body through a physiology of fear, we can begin to do something about it.

It's time to tell our mind: "Hey, let's get back to reality — why are you wearing out the actor with these scripts of anxiety and survival?"

It's time to take back our body and our lives. When we know what we want and are clear about it and listen to our body, it will stop acting as a slave to our stories.

And it can start with something as small as the way we breathe. Breathing rhythmically and with depth can have an incredible effect on our survival syndrome. When we are clear in our thoughts and not clouded by the nonstop scripts our mind is sending to us, we begin to breathe more rhythmically. Our voice begins to change, as well as our facial expressions and our body forms in our abdomen and chest cavities.

Once we understand the secret that we have the power to change the script, huge changes can result. We can overcome our chronic anxiety and our autonomic nervous system no longer needs to be working constantly in the extreme survival syndrome.

If we can arrive at a state where the relationship between our neurotransmitters is balanced, Parkinson's is no longer going to be there as such a strong presence, and we can enter a healthier state of being.

We have to be able to look into our bodies and say, "I know when to stop, I know what to do." Otherwise it's so easy to return to our habits and the forms of Parkinson's.

But if we realize that and know how to communicate with our body through its language, we can keep out the forms of Parkinson's.

"I will change the script and my forms will change!"

"With the help of my brain, my body, and my ability to control my hormones and my feelings, I'll get out of this."

Once we understand that this is what it takes, it becomes such a natural process. We realize immediately where we are headed, and we can say, "Stop."

It takes seconds, not more. As the actor, we analyze the script, we analyze the director, and we react. We say what we have to say through our body, we change our rhythm, our body language, and the forms of our chest and abdomen cavities and our facial expression. And we'll quickly see that our feelings have changed, and we've entered a different script – one that keeps us away from Parkinson's.

Chapter 11

Replacing the Parkinson's Script

Parkinson's disease is a script too – a habitual negative pattern of behavior. And that negative behavior creates the platform where the forms of Parkinson's suit themselves best.

It's become a chronic disease because we have forgotten how to respect our body.

Sometimes, we have to be able to act out the bad or negative script and feel and understand that we are "stuck" – there is no way out of this script. That's when we have to change our body language and forms into a new configuration and look for a way out.

The Parkinson's warrior knows how to change the script, but also knows the bad and the good. The key is to feel how stuck we are being a slave to the forms of Parkinson's and resolve to become a Parkinson's warrior by changing our body forms, movements, and rhythm.

The Academy Awards

We are all actors, and we all win Oscars no matter what we have going on in our lives. Parkinson's sufferers often act "super-Parkinsonian." If we put a camera on ourselves and film how we act, we're the best — all the rest are imitators. Hollywood actors would have so much to learn from us.

So if we can act Parkinson's and win an Academy Award, why can't we do the opposite and say, "I'm going to act like a healthy person." Act healthy until you actually feel healthy. FAKE IT UNTIL YOU MAKE IT. And once you make it, you can say, "I did it – I won another Oscar."

The script that we've received is called "I've Got Parkinson's." But the script that we're going to act out from now on is "I'm a Healthy Person with Parkinson's Symptoms."

Life is a long series of acts — so be the best actor you can. Always be aware of your script and your director. But remember, you are the actor.

And the Oscar goes to...

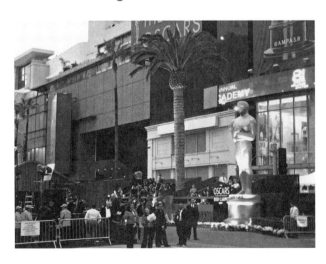

Chapter 12

The Mind: From an Enemy to a True Friend

Until now, we have seen how the mind — with its constant scripts from the past and the future — has ignored the body and done it grievous harm.

But the mind can also be the key in restoring the body to health. Our mind is our true friend when it's in a real communicative relationship with the body. When they are working together, the body feels and gives information and the mind analyzes and finds solutions. When the body and mind interact like a couple in a real relationship, the mind will naturally try to help the body.

Whereas before, the mind was the enemy, now it's a true friend because it's asking the body how it feels and what it wants.

If the body tells us, "I feel heavy," the mind can tell it, "Lighter, lighter" — and all of a sudden we walk in a lighter manner. Or if the body is stuck in a certain situation, the mind can analyze what's going on, explain to the body that it's behaving according to a past script, and say, "We don't need it anymore."

Once the mind and body are able to interact like that with true awareness and communication, then they are on the road to establishing a powerful potential toward rehabilitating and healing the body.

Communicate with the Body

One of the main problems in any relationship between people is communication, and it's the same between the mind and the body.

Using the people analogy, if we have a good physical relationship with our partner, it will be fun, but at a certain time it won't work anymore if we don't have a mental relationship. Likewise, if we connect with someone on a cerebral level, but there's no physical relationship, it also won't work. But if we have both a physical and mental relationship with someone, it's wonderful.

It's the same way with the body and the mind. If the mind dominates and doesn't listen to the body, we are in trouble. And if the body blocks out the good advice that the mind is giving it, it will also result in a failed relationship.

A physically disabled person may fantasize about getting up and walking – and in his mind, he's actually doing it. But when he returns from his fantasy, he's still there in the wheelchair.

Likewise, the body gets lost inside the mind's constant scripts and analysis. It sees that the one speaking and giving the answers is the mind, and the body defers to a one-sided relationship.

But once there's a realization that the mind can't act without the body and the body without the mind, then real progress can be made. *The mind does the thinking and the body does the feeling.*

With Parkinson's, once the body realizes it can't carry on without the mind, and the mind realizes it can't carry on without the body, they start to communicate. And once they communicate, they get answers from each other. Working together in entrainment, they can support each other, listen to one another, and they can begin to change the forms of Parkinson's.

The mind can ask questions and the body can say what it feels. It's the word-versus-sentence paradigm that we talked about earlier. The body realizes that it needs the mind to get the answers to understand how it should behave. And the mind has to pay attention and say, "You have to behave differently. Stop behaving in the past, behave in the present. Change your forms, change your movements, listen to your rhythm, breathe correctly."

When the mind and body work together, and the script is not a Parkinson's script, the mind can tell the body, "See how you feel, see how excited you are? Look how beautifully you've done that."

And the feelings and hormones that are secreted at that point are among the strongest hormones of well-being that we have – they are the hormones of "I can do it," and they are actually the secret to "I can do it."

A Step Back

The excitement and elation that you'll feel over being able to do the exercises in this book and being able to move with fewer Parkinson's symptoms are amazing.

But even with those victories, the mind naturally begins to revert back to the past. The body starts to behave according to its old Parkinsonian habits – old habits are always stronger than the new habits that are built.

The mind reverts back to entering one script after another and doesn't realize that it's going one way and the body another way. The body returns to Parkinson's when the mind isn't united with it.

The body doesn't have a past or future, like the mind does. It has only a present. So if the mind is obsessing about the past or the future, the body is going to behave according to the past or the future.

If the body behaves according to the past, then the past becomes the present. The body can't analyze and doesn't realize it's behaving according to Parkinson's, which is part of the past. The body can only understand it when the mind unites with it and they start to communicate.

This is where the power of the human mind comes in. Yes, as we've learned, it can do damage with its scripts and anxiety. But when it realizes what it's doing and communicates with the body, it can analyze what's happening and tell the body, "No! You're returning to your old habits."

The "Ahhh" Moment

The body speaks through feelings and the greatest word in the body's vocabulary is... "Ahhh."

That happens when the mind explains that the current situation is not the end of the world. The mind can select a script that contains panic, survival, but the mind also has the power to stop and put that script back. "I don't want that script, I want a different one. I don't have to be sick, I can be healthy. I can feel good because I know how to feel bad and I want that habit to change."

Between the body's feeling and the mind's analyzing, we can change the script and change the forms of Parkinson's.

Chapter 13

Percentage of Parkinson's

When we enter our survival syndrome and stay there, it enables an unholy alliance to form. Parkinson's has united with anxiety and the physiology of fear and we've allowed the forms of Parkinson's to take hold.

But are all the symptoms that we're experiencing derived from the Parkinson's? Or are some of them emanating from that fear and the anxiety? We might only have 10% to 15% of what is considered Parkinson's disease. However, due to the reason we've discussed that opened the door for the forms of Parkinson's, we might be manifesting the symptoms of a person with 70% to 80% of the disease.

The Parkinson's we think we have may not be what it seems. If we can learn to put our fear and anxiety aside, we might discover that our level of Parkinson's is not 60% – it's much lower. The entire patient picture is like a puzzle made up of many elements, with Parkinson's being only one.

The problem is that when we go to the doctor, mired deep in our script of anxiety and fear that manifests itself via our Parkinson's body forms and behavior, the doctor will react according to the situation he sees before him. His diagnosis and medication prescription will be based on that heavy-duty Parkinson's patient, not the marginal Parkinson's patient who is exhibiting symptoms derived in part from anxiety and the behavior of fear.

Think of Parkinson's as a big puzzle, a living puzzle. All the people in our past, the stories we tell ourselves, the stories told to us, are just pieces of the puzzle. Every time we take out a piece of that puzzle, the whole puzzle has to reconfigure itself, the whole picture changes. Change the form of one thing and the pieces can no longer fit within the larger puzzle space, and then everything changes.

Parkinson's is really just the name for a puzzle that suits certain situations. If we don't realize that and we rely solely on doctors and medicine, it will undoubtedly get worse. When we feel badly and are in a negative state, we're acting a self-perpetuating script and we wind up deep inside the forms of Parkinson's.

Because of these behavior habits, doctors correctly emphasize the importance of body exercises and physical training as part of any regimen to ward off those Parkinson's forms. But we not only need to take responsibility for our body, we also need to fight to change the script with different behavior.

Then we will see how the puzzle changes and our Parkinson's is different. Then we can see how much or how little Parkinson's we may have. We feel better, we move better, and our mood has changed.

The key is to be able to put the Parkinson's aside, look at and analyze our behavior patterns, and determine what is really causing our symptoms – is it the Parkinson's or is it also our mind? How much Parkinson's do I have and how much is my behavior? How much is Parkinson's and how much anxiety? How much is Parkinson's and how much are the scripts we're acting out?

When we recognize that and are able to change the script to remove the fear and anxiety, then the percentage of Parkinson's can be greatly diminished. We can begin to block out the forms of Parkinson's.

When we regain our confidence, establish a sense of support, and feel good, then the power of Parkinson's loses percentages. It's no longer the same Parkinson's, and we no longer are the same people.

Parkinson's does not know how to behave when we feel good. It only comes out in force when we feel bad, when our script is negative, when we behave Parkinson's and enter its forms.

Once we change the script and the body forms and behave differently, something happens to Parkinson's. And we are freed.

Change your forms. Change your chemistry. Change your puzzle. Change your life!

To be healthy and feel healthy, we need to be aware of all of those aspects of our body, our rhythms, and our movements – and work on it. In the following pages, we will learn a series of exercises that will enable us to make a startling discovery. We don't need to be living in the forms of Parkinson's – we are actually Parkinson's warriors!

A Client Encounter

PERCENTAGE OF PARKINSON'S

I had a client who I hadn't seen in around three months. When I asked him where he had been, he told me that he hadn't come because he was feeling good.

That was a mistake – you need to concentrate on your treatment when you feel good, so you can continue to feel good.

Sure enough, one day he called me in a panic and said he had to see me. He arrived during lunchtime with his wife, and he didn't look good. His leg had some tremors.

"The percentage of my Parkinson's has increased so much," he said in the manner that I had taught him. "It's taking over my life. I can't sit with people anymore, and I've decided to leave my job."

He disclosed that he had recently been to his doctor, who had upped his medication that he was taking from one to three times a day.

"Tell me," I asked. "Have you been abroad lately?"

"Yes, we were in Romania," he answered.

I asked him to tell me about it and he started, "We went to casinos, we had massages, it was so beautiful."

He had started to smile, and I spoke to him.

"Where were you just now?"

"What do you mean?"

"What did you see?"

He told me that he was imagining the casinos and the massage. And from the look in his eyes and on his face, you could tell that the Parkinson's was not there. He had momentarily forgotten about his troubles.

I asked him if he suffered from anxiety and he answered no. I repeated the question and got the same answer.

I asked his wife what he was like at home and she said, "He doesn't stop speaking negatively about what's going to happen to him. He's scared and says all the time, 'Look how I look, look at my face.' He's at the computer all the time googling Parkinson's and what to expect as it gets worse."

I looked at him and said to him, "You see, this has become your script. It's not that the percentage of Parkinson's has become higher. But you've created a script for yourself in which you've begun acting Parkinson's and fearing a negative future and you've become obsessive about it.

"What percentage is Parkinson's and what percentage is you placing your fears and anxieties on top of it?

"That's why when you went to see your doctor, he saw 80% Parkinson's and gave you medication accordingly. It's a mistake! You might only have 25 to 30% Parkinson's and the rest is your mind."

"It true," he said. "I'm living in fear of the future all the time. It's why I don't want to go out or see people. I can't concentrate."

"So let's look at your problem as concentration deficit disorder," I said.

"It's not the Parkinson's but you've entered a stage where your script is titled 'Fear.' And once you're living fear, then you're in your survival syndrome. And once you're there, then you feel abandoned and lost. That's the whole story – you've got it, now get out of it.

"Each time you start living that story, say 'Stop! Is this relevant? Is this true?' Say 'I'm not going to listen to that voice, I'm going to ride a bike instead, I'm going to have a cup of coffee. You'll see, soon you'll feel good and you'll be back going out and meeting people.'"

I told the actor that he can tell the script he was given that it doesn't suit him and he can change it.

SECTION 2

THE EXERCISES

Chapter 14

Introduction to the Exercises: The Body Forms

"When you let go, you let go of your history."
— Alex Kerten

We have learned that Parkinson's patients adjust to the forms, shapes, and behavior of Parkinson's. It's noticeable in the hands, mouths, eyes, breathing patterns, and chest and abdominal cavities. Our act becomes Parkinson's.

If we don't want people to see that something might be wrong with us, we attempt to conceal the symptom or compensate for it. If we have tremors in our hands because of PD, the natural tendency is to hide them. But in doing so, we eliminate a big percentage of our potential for expression by suppressing it.

The irony is that because we don't want anyone to see our symptoms, they become more obvious. We look like we're trying to hide something and it becomes apparent that indeed we are.

Don't Hide, Change!

Instead of trying to hide the Parkinson's symptoms, we need to become aware of our Parkinson's body forms and the scripts that are propelling them forward. Once we do that, we can start changing them into the forms and scripts of a healthy person.

If we want to act out the script of being healthy, then we must learn how to change our body forms and teach them — especially our abdominal and chest cavities — to take on the forms of being healthy. We need to feel and bring back movement within those cavities.

Our eyes, which see our stories and scripts, will begin to see a healthy story, and they will change their expression. Our mouth will change its shape; and our breathing rhythm will change as our body's breathing and rhythm become in step with each other — a state known as *entrainment*.

The Importance of Breathing

Breathing is necessary for every act our body and mind take part in — movement, feelings, and the state of mind we are in. If we're aware of our breathing and its rhythm, we can change our script — *we can change our state of mind through breathing!*

How many times have we been given this advice when we're nervous before a big presentation or performance: "Just take a deep breath, it will be fine."

Breathing controls everything. But we also need to change the look in our eyes. Our script comes from our eyes, and if we're still in that old Parkinson's script, then our breathing and our eyes remain in the old negative entrainment.

With the following exercises, we are going to learn how to change our breathing and rhythms, how to alter our facial expressions and body forms. Then something will begin to take place within our autonomic nervous system, and we'll begin to retake control of our body.

That's the basics of the Gyro-Kinetics method. I have spent decades developing and successfully treating hundreds of patients with Parkinson's. And I'm now going to reveal it to you and explain how to perform these simple yet incredibly effective exercises at home.

But first, we must take a look at our body forms.

Body Forms

Every body form has an effect on our feelings and vice versa, just as our neural network has an effect on our biochemistry, which triggers our feelings.

Our body forms = spirit. So if we can change our spirit, we can change our lives. Our body forms are in charge of everything – our heart, our breathing. Our body forms are energy!

When we leave our balanced state and our survival syndrome takes over, it has an effect on every part of our body through the actions of our autonomic nervous system.

We need to become intimately acquainted with our Parkinson's body forms so when our body forms change, we'll be aware of it. We can then lead ourselves to the most appropriate place where we want to remain.

The moment we feel our forms, we provide our body with pharmacological information. The more medication we take, the less ability we have to do this.

Every morning when we wake up, we should ask our body what it needs and wants. The power of our mind and body is so potent, it will tell us.

Ask ourselves 100 times a day, "What does my body reflect? What is it telling me?"

Be in constant communication with the body forms of Parkinson's.

Do you have back pain? Something is wrong with the movement – the back is stuck.

Feel it! Move the abdominal muscles, enter the pain, enter slow movements. Take out the spirit of the back pain! Let the spirit of the abdomen muscles enter through breathing and moving your back!

Back pain is in most cases due to stuck movements. The body is asking us to change this condition via easy and soft internal movement.

Meeting Our Body

Let's think of the body as being divided into different sections.

Abdominal Cavity

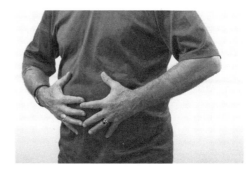

Besides our intelligent digestive system, we also have our abdominal and digestive system muscles. In our abdomen, we find the power of chi (the factory of energy) – the grace and strength we see in a jaguar.

Diaphragm

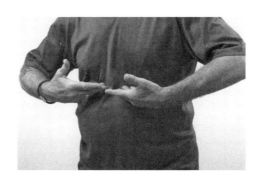

Our diaphragm divides our chest cavity between the lungs and the gastroenterological system – it provides us with our breathing movements and breathing rhythm and is a pathway to our feelings.

Digestive System

If we think about the digestive system, we'll be surprised at how intelligent it is. It receives raw materials, digests them, separates off waste from what the body needs for nourishment, and sends off the desired material to the liver, the heart, the brain, and other organs. Whatever is not required is excreted.

That means there's a tremendous intelligence in our digestive system – it's very aware of the state that our body and mind are in.

If we're in a balanced state, the digestive system has balanced internal movements. If we're in survival syndrome, our digestive system changes immediately – we might get a nervous stomach and diarrhea or feel very constipated.

We have feelings and movements in our digestive system – and we even say it. "I have a gut feeling." "I feel an ache in my belly." "That makes me nauseous."

The Heart

It's not a coincidence that our heart is situated next to our diaphragm, which divides our abdominal cavity and chest cavity. Breathing – taking

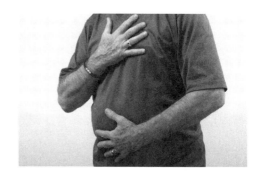

oxygen in and expelling carbon dioxide – is only part of the system. It is actually a matter of feeling, movements, and rhythms based on what state we're in.

It is also a matter of our survival – our heartbeat and our rhythm reflect the feelings we are going through and the script that we are acting.

Therefore, we can control our heartbeat and change our feelings through breathing exercises – it's a very important part of life that we have control over!

Through breathing, and specifically through our diaphragm, we can fine-tune our heartbeat.

Through atmospheric pressure, our lungs inflate and deflate and determine the way we breathe. It's not through our muscles. This means that the rhythm of the diaphragm and the state it's in also has control over our heart.

But our heart is not just a muscle – we feel in our heart as well. Most songs are written about the heart, and heartache. The heart is a center of emotion.

According to what we feel in our heart, information is passed on to our autonomic nervous system, which is in charge of all of our body systems. If we're in survival mode, our systems enter that syndrome too. But if we're balanced, our systems function normally.

With every feeling we have, our abdomen and chest cavity change shape – there are different forms for anger, hurt, happiness – they change shapes every split second according to our feelings.

It's quite astounding, but it's true. Through being aware of our breathing and our heartbeat (how our diaphragm and chest cavity are feeling), we can control our autonomic nervous system!

Face and Eyes

Our face and our facial expressions communicate the script that we pass on to and from the brain through our expressions and body language.

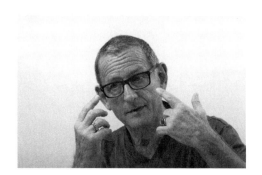

We use our eyes, of course, to see.

But when we look into someone else's eyes, we not only have a window into their soul, we can also see what kind of state that person is in – sad, happy, pained, confused.

Just like our chest and abdominal cavities, our eyes change forms according to every feeling that we have.

In addition, our eyes take us places. If I ask you how your vacation in London was, your eyes will take you to London as you describe your experiences at Piccadilly Circus and Covent Garden. You are there, and I am now in the background.

Our stories and scripts do not originate in our brain, they start in our eyes. We see our story, like the cliché says, unfold before our very eyes and we transmit that picture to the brain.

Our eyes see and transmit to our brain what they want. This is important because the scripts that our brain processes begin with the eyes. The eyes are constantly giving the scripts to our mind that are passed on to our body.

With the onset of Parkinson's, we see with our eyes where we could be headed. The more people with Parkinson's that we see and the more we read about the prospects of our deterioration, the more we enter the shapes and body forms of Parkinson's – because we see it in our eyes and act it through our mind and body.

Mouth

We speak with our mouth, give rhythm with our mouth, inhale and exhale with our mouth when we need to express ourselves or need to be in 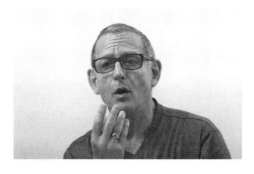 control of our breathing while running, singing, or performing some other physical activity.

What our eyes see is actualized by what we say and how we breathe. As our eyes change according to what we see, our mouth also changes. They work together, making up a natural audiovisual system.

Hands

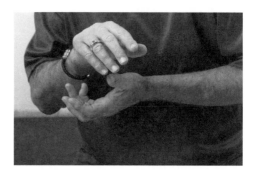

Our hands are used for holding, but they also give us rhythm and expression, and help us think better. Just recall all the times we use our hands to help us recover a memory, make a point in discussion, or accentuate a statement.

Our hands make forms and help us remember what we wanted to see with our eyes. They push our memory along and spark new scenarios.

If we stop using our hands because we don't want to show tremors, and we don't speak with expression enhanced by hand movements, it has an effect on our memory and it has an effect on our expression. We end up with a frozen face, frozen shoulders, and a frozen personality.

Chapter 15

Exercises for Life

Gyro-Kinetics exercises are not simply a series of activities that can be pulled out from time to time when we're not feeling good and then put away — they have to become a way of life.

If we're going to learn a new language because we're moving to a foreign country, we have to immerse ourselves in it 24 hours a day. If we want to divorce ourselves from Parkinson's, it's the same as divorcing ourselves from a spouse. We can't do it part-time.

Although we can't divorce our habits, we can change the forms of our habits. And that's what we're going to do.

We're going to learn how to breathe rhythmically and use our facial expressions and hands. We're going to learn about the art of movement and its importance in blocking out the forms of Parkinson's.

We're not going to practice and then go back to Parkinson's habits. No way! We're going to practice, be aware of what we're doing and how it's changing us. We're going to integrate what we learn into our daily lives, which will enable us to say NO to Parkinson's.

Keep these exercises close to the heart while doing everything else in life – at home, at work, talking to people, going to the movies. The goal is to feel good 24 hours a day, not just while doing the exercise – and believe me, you will feel good doing the exercises!

We don't want to return to our previous state consisting of the habits and scripts of Parkinson's. But unfortunately, that's the sad story of the whole world, not just PD patients. We go somewhere, do something transcendent, and then we go back home to our old habits… and it's all gone.

We need to ask ourselves: "Are these good behavior habits or bad behavior habits? Do I want them to continue or go away? If I want them to go away, why am I always returning to the old habits?"

The answer is because we are brainwashed. So the solution is: "Brainwash yourselves in the opposite direction, toward what you really want."

Working on these exercises 30 to 40 minutes a day will train us that even small movements will cause huge changes. When we move our frame even slightly, it affects other parts of our body. The more we change our forms by moving our body and facial expressions, the more we change our tree trunk, causing our tremors and chaotic rhythms to change accordingly.

Smile at the tremors, and keep doing it until you find the new forms! It is hard work, but with time you will notice a change and a decrease in the tremors.

When we begin to breath rhythmically, dance, conduct, and learn how to move, our autonomic nervous system will start to work differently. It's all a matter of awareness and realizing there is a place where Parkinson's is weak! *There is a mid-rhythm between the fast chaos of dyskinesia and the slow gait of freezing.* At the extremes, Parkinson's is strong – but when we breathe rhythmically and move in rhythm heading toward our home alpha state base, then where is the Parkinson's? It's been replaced by a sense of confidence and a spirit of feeling good.

Once we look at our body this way, we see that the body provides most of the answers for us. And we'll understand how to enter our body and change its rhythm and shapes. We'll realize that we haven't been breathing with our abdomen properly, we've been breathing with our throat. We've been using a third of our lung capacity – a sure sign that we're in survival syndrome.

Once we learn how to move and breathe correctly and with confidence, we'll see a change in our facial expressions and in our eyes. And once we change our facial expressions and are aware of our eyes, we'll discover that the script that we've been stuck in has been released – we've been liberated.

Stop Thinking

This is a very important part of the process – stop thinking! Enter your body!

We need to see the body as a personality, a being, and ask him what it wants. Don't bring stories and scripts with you – just listen and be there. Close your eyes and breathe into your body and feel what's going on there. There's always movement – movement of sadness or happiness, movement of disease, of being healthy and of uncertainty.

Our movements and hormones = feelings, and you need to enter those feelings and breathe those feelings. Remain there and keep asking your body: What do you want, what are you trying to tell me?

Let's get to work. You'll be amazed to discover how the body answers you.

EXERCISE 1: Breathing

WHY THIS IS IMPORTANT

Breathing is the most wonderful thing we can do with our body. Whether we're speaking, walking, or sitting, our breathing dictates the rhythm for that action.

Feelings have their own rhythm that determines how we breathe. If we're happy, we breathe the rhythm of happiness – deep and satisfying. If we're nervous, we breathe the rhythm of nervousness – short, clipped breaths. With every act and every feeling we have, breathing is parallel.

Our diaphragm – which divides the abdominal cavity from the chest cavity – is the secret of breathing. When we inflate our lungs, the diaphragm goes down and when we exhale, the diaphragm goes up, resulting in inflating and deflating abdominal movements. Because the heart is situated close to the diaphragm, the breathing movements have an effect on the heart as well.

The effects of Parkinson's restricts the diaphragm's ability to do its job, and here I will show you how to regain full control of your breathing and speech potential.

DIAPHRAGM – The diaphragm is the key to our breathing movement, our breathing rhythm, and it can help the body express its "feelings."

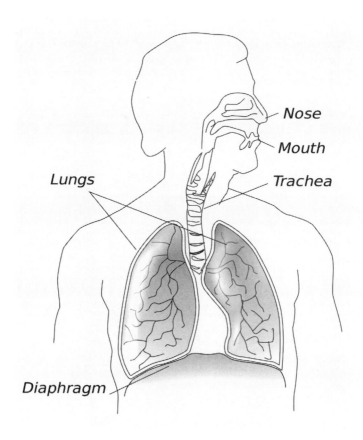

Nose

Mouth

Lungs

Trachea

Diaphragm

● *EXERCISE*

You can do this exercise standing or sitting, with your eyes closed or open. The only thing you need to do is CONCENTRATE.

Concentrate = Meditate. Be aware of what you're doing and stop the scenario (the thoughts and stories in your mind) that you're stuck in. Instead breathe deeply through your mouth and enter your abdominal cavity and remain there.

Breathe into it – you will realize an outstanding world of movements in your abdominal cavity.

Think about what's happening there – What movements do I have (fast, slow, stimulating, or relaxing)?

Inhale again and feel the flow of the river going into your abdominal cavity. Feel how your breathing goes down. Feel what's happening – how your abdomen is inflating, deflating, and the movements you have within your abdominal cavity.

Your feelings should change too. Feel the excitement. You start to feel hormones kicking in – you feel good, you feel confidence and energy.

Continue breathing through your abdomen into your chest cavity and feel how through your abdominal breathing you're inflating your chest cavity.

You'll suddenly begin to feel how your ribs start to become more springy, more supple – and your heartbeat starts to go down and your heart is inflating. Your diaphragm, which has been constricted, is now open and working to its full capacity.

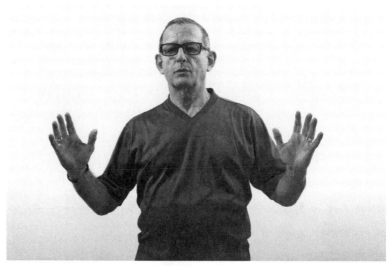

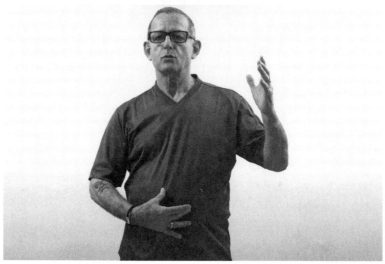

You feel more power in your heart, it is becoming stronger. You will hear the language of your heart. The heart speaks all the time – whether you feel confidence, depression, joy – you feel it in your heart and in your rhythmic breathing.

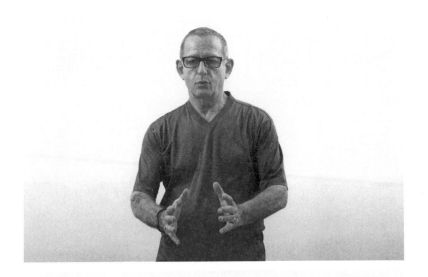

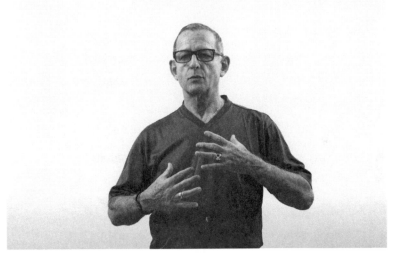

By being aware of your different rhythmic breathing, you are able to change the movements within your chest cavity and bring more space to the heart. And by changing these forms within your abdomen and chest cavity you've changed the scenario.

You will notice that once you breathe correctly and with confidence, you will change your facial expressions as well. What you are seeing in your mind, through your eyes whether open or closed, has been changed. You will see that the scenario you were stuck in has been freed. You are in harmony.

And this is the most important part of the process: stop thinking! Just be there.

Because each scenario you bring in is a neural stimulation taking place between your past experiences and future scenarios. Stop your thoughts, be aware of your body language and forms, and remain in the present. Only then can you decide what you want to feel and look like in the future.

Don't bring in another script and another story. Do you feel good? Do you feel healthier? Remain there!

The best teacher for breathing is a singer – a good singer like Ella Fitzgerald or Frank Sinatra.

Put some music like that on, close your eyes, feel the way you breathe into your abdomen, and listen to the singer. Breathe with the phrasing of the singer – you will see that he breathes rhythmically, sometimes picking it up, sometimes slowing it down. Breathe with the singer as if you are the singer.

What happens? You stimulate your brain and your scenario becomes you as the singer. His story, the rhythm of the song, and the potential of the singer enter into you. And your own story changes, thus making changes within your nervous system. You will be surprised by the effects you will feel in your body and speech.

ALEX'S ENCOURAGEMENT

When you are not balanced in your breathing rhythms, you are in a state of mental and physical chaos. You've created a scenario based on your survival syndrome.

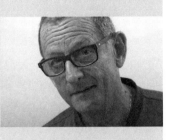

Once you are aware of it, you can change your scenario by consciously changing your breathing and rhythm. Your body begins to work in harmony... and then the miracle takes place. You can change your state of mind through your breathing and body awareness. Speak with your body daily like you would speak to a loved one in your family.

THOUGHT FOR THE DAY

Thinking is our problem. Awareness is what we need. So don't think, be aware!

WHY IT WORKS

When we think, we secrete hormones. The way we secrete them has an effect on our physiology. So if we make some physiological changes – meaning **if we focus on our body language and forms, our body movement, rhythm, breathing, and our facial expressions – it will have an effect on our biology and biochemistry**, those neurotransmitters that when functioning correctly are creating our middle home base. This, in turn, will influence our psychology – the ongoing conversation between our script, our director, and our body.

EXERCISE 2: Hands and Facial Expressions

WHY THIS IS IMPORTANT

In general, people with Parkinson's are not very expressive, and in fact, they tend to freeze their facial expressions and hand movements.

They put a mask on their face and don't move their hands in an attempt to conceal their Parkinson's. That's why in many cases when they express themselves, it's unclear if they're angry, happy, or excited. As a result, a lot of mixed messages are passed and confusion abounds – spouses get annoyed; friends and family think they don't care.

Frozen facial expressions are very Parkinsonian. So is keeping an iron curtain around feelings. But through acting out animated facial expressions, you can break through that wall.

If you're not aware of your facial expressions and don't exercise them at every given moment, they could be lost forever. If you don't use it, you will lose it.

Whatever you are thinking, your mouth and eyes act to reflect that script. If you're thinking Parkinson's and anxiety, then you act Parkinson's and anxiety. Facial expressions help you enter a new story. So, it's time to change the act – and start expressing yourself!

Feelings are one of the most powerful tools you have. If you don't express them, don't communicate with them, and keep them stuck inside, they can lead to chronic disease. If you express them, they can contribute immeasurably to rehabilitation efforts. Once you understand that you need to communicate between your hands, face, and body, you'll discover that your body speaks to you through feelings and information.

The body expresses itself through feelings, body language, and forms. And if you're not aware that the body has its personal language, then it's difficult to communicate with it. Communicating with your body should be like talking to your best friend.

● *EXERCISE*

Facial Expression

Put on some soothing, rhythmic music with a good singer and begin to listen and breathe along with the rhythm of the song.

Start to imitate the singer, let your head go loose, get your face moving. You can also imitate one of the instruments if you prefer. Be part of the song, breathe in and out – it's very important! Change your facial expressions according to your feelings generated by the song. Feel free to sing along out loud and belt out the song.

Listen to each song and make the facial expression of the singer as you act out the song based on the lyrics and his vocal intonations – or make the facial expression of how you think a conductor would look as he orchestrates the swelling music coming out of the speakers.

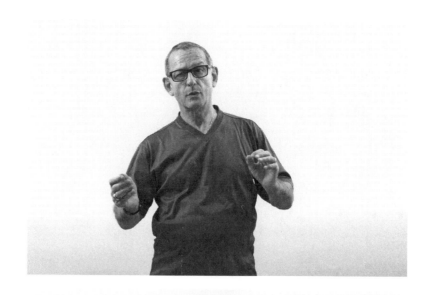

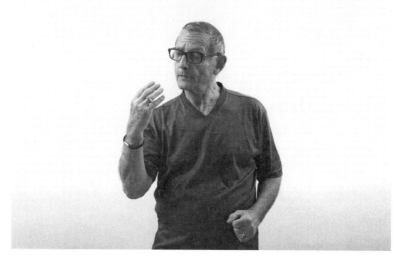

Try to use your entire arsenal: eyebrows, mouth, teeth, forehead, jaw, and even your nose. Feel where you're stuck, feel your habit, and then feel the singer. How does he sing? How does he relate to his feelings? Let go – let your face open up.

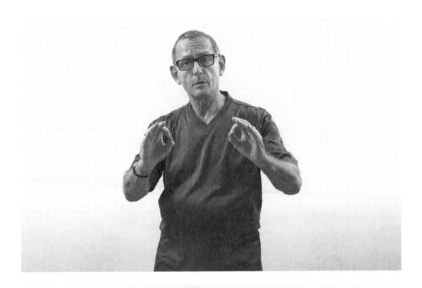

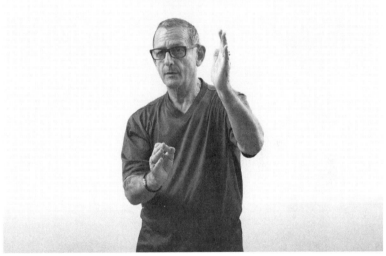

Keep changing the expressions – change the emotions. Change the song too! Switching the song to one with a different rhythm will enable a greater scope of facial expressions and enable you to change along with the emotions oozing out of the song.

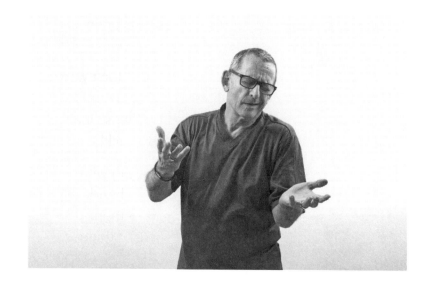

Feel how the face changes, the mouth opens and closes, the eyes go up and down. Work with the feelings and change the expression – Be different!

Keep practicing until it becomes subconscious behavior and an automatic part of your life.

Hands

Once your face is loose and you're comfortable changing your facial expression, remember your hands. Hands are not only for holding, they are also for the expression of rhythm and for aiding our memory.

When we want to recall something, we often make forms with our hands – these forms remind us and stimulate our memory. The hand aids our brain. If we don't remember something, our hands take us there. Before we even speak, our hands make motions and tell us in advance what is happening, while our brain is still processing the information.

So if we stop using our hands because we don't want people to see our tremors, or if we can't use our hands because they are tight and stiff, what happens? It affects our memory and our expression. We are stuck!

Move your hands in a rhythmic fashion along with the music. Interpret the song through your hands and translate the music through your movements. Be spontaneous and improvise – the important thing is that your hands are reacting to the music.

Try to do it at the same time as you work on your facial movements. You'll find a new world of expression opening up that had been closed because of Parkinson's and because of your scripts of anxiety.

Keep moving your hands in different forms as the music passes through different phases. Remember to breathe rhythmically and to enter the song. Become one with the music, and your hands will take on a life of their own.

ALEX'S ENCOURAGEMENT

Once we know how to
control our scripts, we can
maneuver our body and
our feelings like playing
a piano. We feel anxiety?
We can stop it. We feel
tremors? We know how
to limit them. We can feel what is happening to
us and prevent it until it becomes an automatic
process that we don't have to think about anymore.

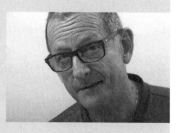

Speak to yourself regularly. Speak with your body.
What do you feel? What is your message? The
mind communicates through sentences. The body
communicates through feelings.

THOUGHT FOR THE DAY

When you want to attract health into your life,
make sure your other attractions don't contradict
your desires. You cannot experience the feelings
of health and happiness unless you invite them in
through persistent thought and action.

EXERCISE 3: Conducting

Why This Is Important

Conducting really means movement. It's all about self-expression, changing your body forms, your breathing patterns, and your facial expressions.

Instead of speaking with words, you are speaking and communicating through your body.

The more you do this exercise – the more you move your hands and arms, change you facial expressions, and breathe differently – you will realize how much you had entered into chronic, habitual Parkinson's behavior and how much you can change that behavior!

Conducting enables you to open up those body forms blocked by Parkinson's and your own scenario and reintroduces you and your body to a different phase of movement. You will become one with the music and you will forget the Parkinson's story – that fear of being seen, of hiding your hands so people don't see your tremors, of pressing your face so it becomes stone.

Conducting is all about rhythm and feeling and expression – it's the antithesis of Parkinson's behavior. It's virtually impossible to remain in your body form and Parkinson's breathing patterns when you conduct – you have to leave Parkinson's. The more you conduct, the less Parkinson's is around.

Control means not having control. With Parkinson's, you are always trying to control your symptoms. With conducting, you don't want – or need – control. You simply flow. The orchestra or band plays, the singer sings, and you let it wash over your body, mind, and soul. Control is the ability to let go, and letting your movements be as they should be – natural and unforced.

When you conduct, you will be amazed at how liberated you will feel.

● *EXERCISE*

The key to conducting is feeling like you're in charge of the music – the band and the singer. Without you, they will not make their beautiful music.

Choose music according to your mood. It should be rhythmic. Your body will tell you what your mood is – it knows whether you want something upbeat or relaxing. You might want Broadway or Sinatra, or disco or marching music or soothing classical music. It doesn't matter. What matters is how you feel about it.

Put on the music and stand in the room with some space to enable you to move around. It's better to say that there are no rules to conducting, your body will tell you the rules. But move your arms in a rhythmic pattern, relax your facial muscles. Be aware of your breathing, your hands, your legs, and at the same time, let them go without thinking about them.

If you change your body movements and facial expressions often, then changes will also take place in the Parkinson's behavior, so *always* change your

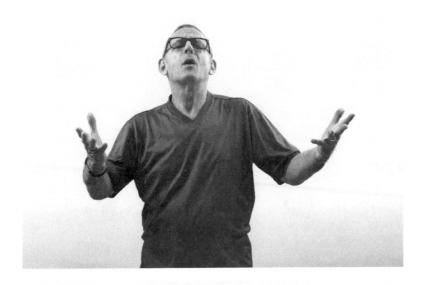

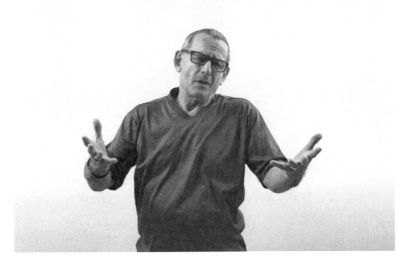

movements and body forms when conducting. Don't just do the same moves – vary them. Maybe raise your hands higher, use more of a flourish – if you feel like dancing along, go ahead!

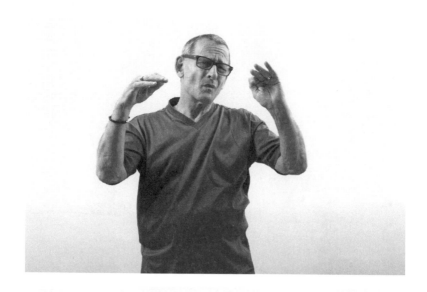

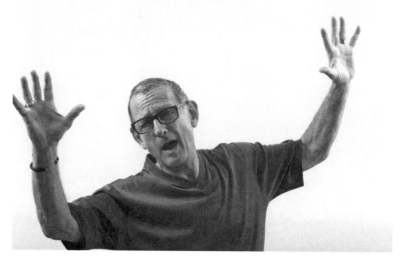

And all of a sudden, you will become a conductor. You will become a warrior, filled with confidence and an internal rhythm that has been robbed by Parkinson's. You'll begin to walk more like you used to before, or in a different style rather than the Parkinson's way of walking.

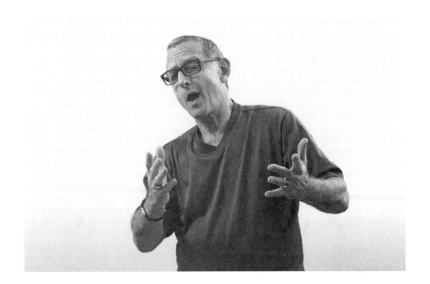

You can do this exercise, even if you have difficulty standing. You can sit, breathe, change your facial expressions – *stop* thinking about your Parkinson's and think about the music.

Start from where you can – move with your face, move with your breathing – and you'll see, you'll begin to feel better.

If you have tremors in your hands, don't try to stop them, but instead, try to bring a rhythm into them. You'll feel very hard, very stuck – you'll think that you can't do it.

But feel that sensation of hardness, being stuck – feel what's happening inside you and say to yourself, "How can it be easier? How can I be lighter? How can I change my rhythm?"

You'll see that something beautiful starts to happen. Your body is your friend – it's saying, "I'm going to help you, I'm going to be with you, I'm your best friend, I'm listening to what's happening to you."

Slowly, you'll see that something is changing in your mind and in your body.

ALEX'S ENCOURAGEMENT

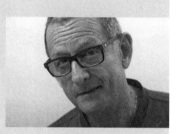

Bring conducting into other facets of your life. Conduct while you speak, move while you speak, change your facial expression while you speak. You might still have tremors but with time, those tremors will change. You'll discover that your breathing, body movements, and facial expressions are in sync with each other – in what we've learned is called entrainment. Instead of the chaotic rhythms you've been experiencing, your Parkinson's will become more systematic and more entrained into a healthy form of movement.

THOUGHT FOR THE DAY

Conducting is being one with the music. If you stop thinking and enter that world, you will also become one with the world.

WHY IT WORKS

All life is a matter of balance, of being in the middle rhythmically, biochemically, and movement-wise. Some people call it the yin and yang of body and soul. It's our home base, our sense of physical and spiritual well-being. Knowing our middle state is one of the secrets of life.

Once we leave our middle for good and move toward an extremity, there can be a grave price to be paid. That's where we wear ourselves out – it's where the term *burned out* comes from. And that's where we become "stuck." We are not aware that our body language – our caved-in chest, our stooped posture – is calling out to us for help.

EXERCISE 4: Conducting Inward/Internal Massage

WHY THIS IS IMPORTANT

When you enter the spirit of Parkinson's, you are no longer moving rhythmically. Your springs and joints are stuck. Your neck, your shoulders, and your back are constantly stiff and you can't move them well. You need an internal massage – if something like that existed. Luckily it does – and it's called conducting inward.

When you conduct internally, you feel the inner movements of your body even if they are stuck. By entering inward and giving yourself an internal massage, you'll see that all your body forms are changing. Internal conducting enables you to cleanse yourself and bring about positive movements.

Movement equals massage. What you will experience is a rhythmic movement massage – a personal massage sparked by the music that enters into you. As opposed to you conducting an orchestra outwardly, the music conducts your internal body forms.

If you feel stiffness in your body and have a difficult time moving certain areas, internal conducting will do wonders to release you and provide a refreshing and invigorating endeavor.

● *EXERCISE*

When you conducted outwardly, you synched yourself with the spirit of the orchestra, the composer, and the singer, and you changed your breathing, facial expressions, body forms, and movements according to the rhythm of the music.

Without realizing it, you received the musical medication of movement, expression, and breathing. It was beautiful, because it taught you that that you can behave differently – the music is always changing so you can also change along with it. You don't have to stay in your Parkinson's patterns, you have the ability to change the scenario with the help of the music and the rhythm and by becoming aware of your body forms.

Now we want to try something a little different. It's time to turn inward and heal yourself.

Put on soothing music that does not necessarily include the steady rhythms required for outward conducting. But it should have a rhythm that can help you regulate your breathing and your movements. No marching band music here, just a piece you like that can take you to a positive place.

Lie down in a comfortable position on your back. Close your eyes and try to empty your mind. Don't think about anything, breathe rhythmically.

Then, start to enter inward. Take a leisurely journey through your body – to your chest, your ribs, vertebrae,

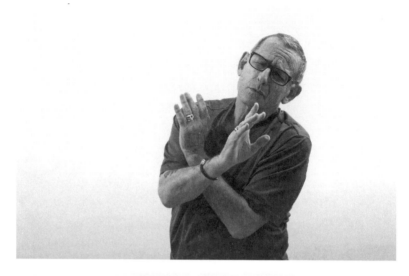

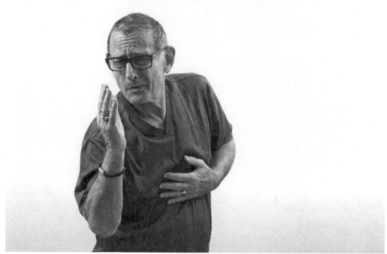

your buttocks, and your pelvis. Try to linger at each stop along way, concentrate on how each part of your body feels, and be aware of its movement or lack of movement.

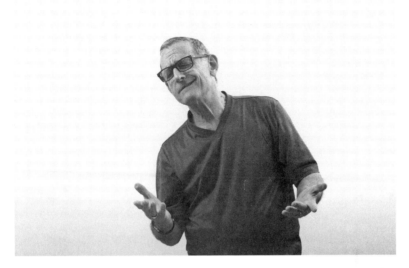

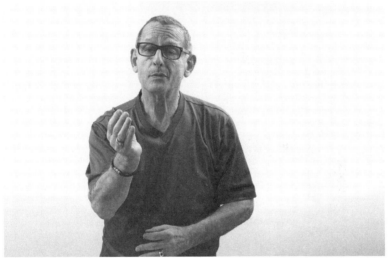

Be aware of how your feet are adjacent to the floor and move them. Notice how your knees are in contact with your legs and their connection to your buttocks and hips. Move them and you'll see that your abdomen

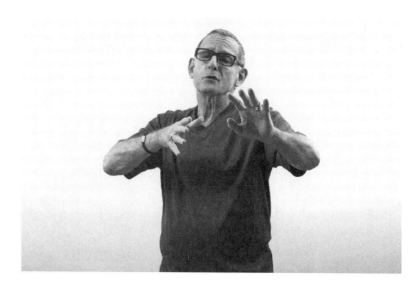

starts to work as well. Try to release your vertebrae and note how it affects your neck and your head.

You will realize suddenly that everything is starting to become lighter and looser – your feet, knees, buttocks, abdominal cavity, neck, and shoulders.

Then try the same movements while standing. By entering inward, your body forms have changed and a healthy spirit has entered instead of a Parkinson's spirit.

There's a guiding principle for students of martial arts that is relevant to internal conducting: if you want to think, stop thinking. Stopping your thoughts is the key – don't bring in any more scenarios. You don't want to think about anything now – feel your body and find out what it wants. Give your body the respect and attention it deserves. It will respond by saying "thank you."

So stop thinking and have a good internal body massage through movement awareness.

ALEX'S ENCOURAGEMENT

The object is to feel good – and internal conducting makes you feel good.

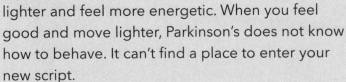

Once you feel good, you feel healthier. And when you feel healthier, you don't walk old or stuck; you walk younger and easier and you look lighter and feel more energetic. When you feel good and move lighter, Parkinson's does not know how to behave. It can't find a place to enter your new script.

THOUGHT FOR THE DAY

My bank account was getting bigger and bigger, but my body was getting stiffer and stiffer. Forget your bank account and pay attention to your body. Will you be happier with a big bank account or a healthy body? With a healthy body, you can decide much more astutely what to do with your bank account.

WHY IT WORKS

The mind needs to understand that it can't live without the body – and the body needs to understand that it can't live without its needs being explained and interpreted by the mind. They must always work together.

When the script accessed from the brain is from the past, the mind and body begin living in the past. But the mind has the ability and the power to say, "No, this isn't correct. I don't want to be in the past anymore. I want to be in the present with the body. The body may have Parkinson's now but I'm going to change the script – I'm not going to listen to the past emanating from my past – those rules that came from my father, my teacher, from God. I don't care anymore. I'm going to be in the present."

EXERCISE 5: Art of Movement/Free Dancing

WHY THIS IS IMPORTANT

Dancing is an expression of improvised movement.

There's a big difference between classical music and jazz. A classical piece is written down and played the same way year after year. With jazz, you'll never play a song the same way twice – it's always different. It's the same with free dancing.

Life is actually one big dance, and free dancing is life. You are dancing with every action and reaction that you have, and the dance changes according to every situation you are confronted with.

Dancing and acting go together hand in hand, so in essence, you dance all the time, without realizing it – whether you're waiting in line at a movie or meeting a bank clerk for a loan. Everything is a dance and everything is acting.

When you dance, you are actually changing your body forms all the time. It all depends on the rhythm, the story in your mind, and the feelings and emotions it gives you.

Some people think that dancing is doing the salsa or the cha-cha. They say, "OK, we're going to teach people with Parkinson's to tango!"

There's nothing wrong with that and if it expands the body's repertoire of movements, it's beneficial. But what is really beneficial is free dancing – taking the music and make an art out of movement.

With free dancing, you can gain a wide-ranging repertoire of movements that give you the ability to get in and out of certain situations. This will expand the body's capabilities, make you more limber, help you find your rhythm, and regain your balanced state. It also feels great!

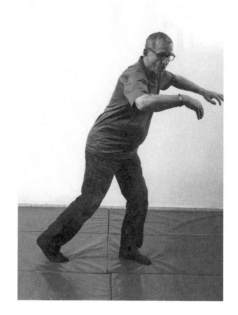

● *EXERCISE*

Take any piece of music – upbeat rhythmic or calming background music – and begin to move. The key is to get all of your body involved in the movement. It doesn't really matter how you express

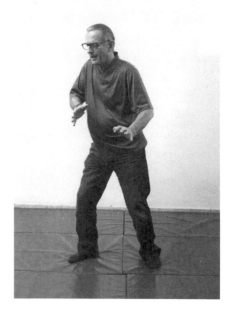

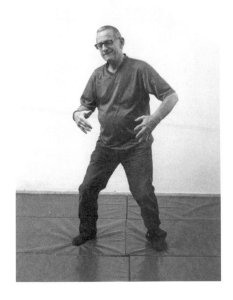

yourself as long as you express yourself!

Without being too conscious of it, notice how your movements are all connected – from your feet and legs on up through your buttocks, your abdomen, your hands, and your facial expressions.

Now, feel what's happening in your vertebrae, in your shoulder blades, how they're loosening and changing shape. You are getting to the root, you are getting to the basics. Be aware!

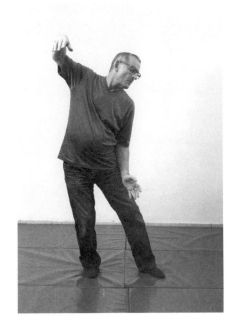

That's dancing! And all of a sudden, you'll start to do it automatically without thinking. When you let go and enter into full movements and expressive movements, your body takes over – and you no longer have to think!

Then, after a few minutes, change the music! When you alter the mood and the rhythm of the music, you'll begin to change your body movements and notice new avenues of expression.

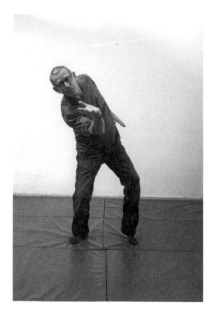

Let the song and the singer wash over you. Translate the music into movements and work on combinations of movements.

Become intimately acquainted with the different rhythms and enter into them – not only on the beat rhythmically, but against the beat of the music in a nonrhythmic manner – you can express yourself however you want. That's the beauty of free dancing, there's no way to do it incorrectly.

You're going to get stimulated. Sometimes, when we're stimulated, it feels good. And sometimes you get stimulated so much, you enter into a state in which you feel that you are losing control. In that case, slow rhythms calm you and bring you toward your alpha state of contentment. Try to use a combination of these

different rhythms and make as many body forms as
you can.

Free dancing means entering from one body form
into another – from one rhythm into another – from
one state of being, one heartbeat, and one breath into
another. You are changing your state of mind and your
body language.

What you learn from free dancing is that you don't have
to stay in the same place. You can dance – and move
– differently. Listen to your body, listen to the rhythm,
your breathing – see what your eyes reflect, because
the eyes reflect the scenario that we have given.

If the dance is sad, then you reflect sadness outward in
your eyes. So when you change the dance, your eyes
also change. You can change the sadness – it's changed
along with your dance.

You can dance sadness, happiness, confidence, anger –
and along with them, you learn the different body forms
that come with them. Then you can decide how you
want to dance your life.

Change the dance, and you change the spirit.

ALEX'S ENCOURAGEMENT

People with Parkinson's
have learned how to
dance only one way – it's
a stiff, limiting array of
movements that take away
your self-confidence and
instruct you to stay within
your new restrictive boundaries of movement.

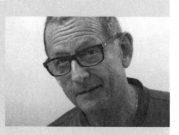

But if in reality, you can dance in many ways, and
it can lead you to change your movements, why
should you choose the Parkinson's way? The key
is to remain in that state – whether you're walking
through an airport, speaking to a client, or getting
coffee at Starbucks. Dance your way through! Don't
return to Parkinson's!

THOUGHT FOR THE DAY

If you know how to dance your way through life,
then that dance becomes your act and your way
of life. You can dance a healthy dance, a rhythmic
dance. And once you do that, your brain will
get the idea that you don't have to dance the
Parkinson's dance anymore.

EXERCISE 6: The Spring Theory

WHY THIS IS IMPORTANT

One way to view the body is as an interrelated set of muscular springs. We have springs in our elbows, mouth, eyes, heart, diaphragm, chest, ribs, and vertebrae.

When we discover that our movements are stuck, limited, or causing pain, we can try to break out of it using the spring metaphor. To do so, we can define four states of being or statuses for our springs:

- BALANCED SPRING: working well, contracting and expanding. The muscular system's contractions, flexing, its neural impulses reaching it from the brain and its blood supply are all working in harmony and coherence.

- SEMI-CONTRACTED SPRING: A spring that is stuck in a certain place, perhaps due to a blocked neural impulse or blood supply. It may be manifested in a stiff neck or shoulders, constricted abdomen or chest, or incomplete movement of one of the limbs.

- CONTRACTED SPRING: A spring that is really stuck and loses its ability to move. It can show itself in tremors, spasms, or in freezing.

- FALLEN SPRING: The muscles lose their spring potential – called *muscular hypo tonus*. There is no movement.

The spring metaphor is also relevant not just for the muscular and cardiovascular systems, but the respiratory and digestive systems as well. They all work like springs, with the ability to contract and return to their balanced original size and shape.

When the springs are working together in a balanced state, it helps all of the body systems work more efficiently to maintain maximum movement potential. Muscles affected by Parkinson's, however, have difficulty returning to their original size and tone when in use.

We can use the four states of the spring to stimulate the muscular system to bring the contraction size and tone back to its normal state and head toward a balanced spring potential.

● *EXERCISE*

How can we stimulate a spring that is stuck in a certain place to work again? Try this exercise.

Put on some midtempo music, close your eyes, and enter your body. Feel where you're stuck and breathe into it – bring movement into it. Try to be lighter, more bouncy... more springy.

Become a "skeleton" and try to move all your joints from top to bottom. Then try to move your muscles. Let your body decide which movements to make.

Remember to breathe rhythmically with each movement you make. Be aware of each part of your

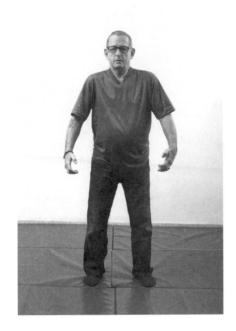

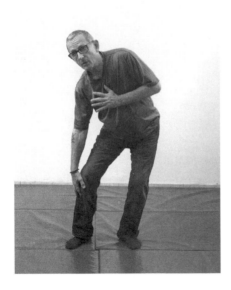

body and make "fine-tuning repairs" while moving to the beat of the music.

Think of your body as a series of springs that need to bounce back into place.

Concentrate on your shoulders – move them around in a circular motion and feel the muscles spring back and forth. Then repeat in the opposite direction. Do this for a minute or two and feel how the shoulders begin to loosen up and become more limber.

Try the same thing with your neck. Move it slowly in a circular motion, first going one way and then another. Feel how the neck muscles begin to relax and regain their form.

Do the same with the mouth. Move it around in different shapes, getting it out of its frozen form with fallen springs. Put the spring back into it.

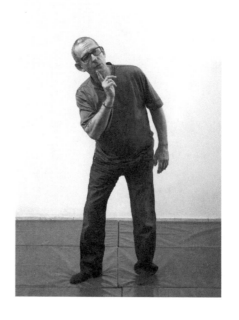

Continue down to your arms, moving them outstretched in a circular fashion, like you're a windmill. Feel them spring back to life. Clench your hands and release them. Do it repeatedly.

If it's more conducive, use the conducting exercise again to engage your upper torso in constant movement. And employ the art of movement to improvise with your legs as you dance around. Breathe deeply, get the springs in your abdomen and

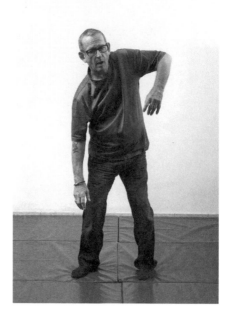

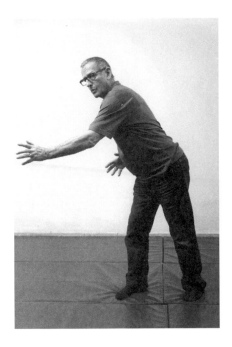

chest to expand and contract and feel them open up where they were constricted.

Slowly you will feel a change. It will hurt, but embrace the feeling, and soon that feeling will change. It may be a different kind of pain, or the pain may subside. In either case, something is happening. And you'll notice the springs loosening up and slowly begin to contract and expand like they used to.

You can stimulate your brain to train your body to behave in a new way. Whereas before you were being given the script of being stuck with fallen springs, you can replace the script with a new one.

Your neck and shoulders will loosen up, the forms of your abdomen and chest will expand, and your limbs will become unstuck.

On days when you feel stuck, in pain, and headed for despair, try thinking of your body as this system of springs. Concentrate on returning them from fallen to balanced springs, and then you too will be headed for your balanced state.

ALEX'S ENCOURAGEMENT

Life is an ongoing jam session – between being happy and sad, angry and letting go, between being healthy and diseased. The jam session improvises in its search for that middle 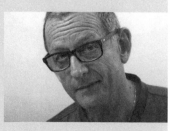 ground. Once you find it, you then have the ability to stay there and keep jamming.

THOUGHT FOR THE DAY

There's a saying in Japanese that when you're balanced in your yin and yang, you're in a state of agelessness. Why? Because you're rhythmic, and you're springy.

WHY IT WORKS

We think that feeling good is achieved from getting a raise, going shopping, walking down a red carpet. But don't buy it. It's not true.

The real meaning of feeling good is entering our body and our body responding by saying, "Thank you, I feel good."

That means we feel good in our abdomen, our chest, our heart, and in the way we breathe.

EXERCISE 7: The Body Player

WHY THIS IS IMPORTANT

You've learned how to conduct inward and outward, to massage your body internally, and how to use the art of movement. They have enabled you to free yourself from the body forms of Parkinson's and have showed you that when your breathing and rhythm are in sync, you are able to change your Parkinson's script.

As you've learned, rhythm, feeling, and expression are the antithesis of the stuck behavior of Parkinson's. And the more you work your rhythm and feeling and express yourself, the less Parkinson's is present because it doesn't know how to be there when you're feeling good.

But you also have to cope with human nature. It's so easy for you to fall back into your Parkinsonian habits, because old habits are much more powerful than the new healthful habits you've been picking up. When conducting or free dancing are no longer providing enough of a challenge, or are not doing enough for you anymore to unblock your constricted and stuck abdomen, chest, hands, and face, it is time to try to become a body player.

The body player exercise takes everything you've learned about movement and getting in touch with your body and brings it to the limits of expression. You've led the orchestra, imitated the singer, and improvised your movements to the music. Now you're going to become the instruments of the song – an exercise that will open up the body and the soul to new avenues that have yet to be explored.

You're going to become a member of a finely tuned, interconnected combo in which everything must mesh and work together or it won't work at all.

The ultimate liberation from restriction is just around the corner.

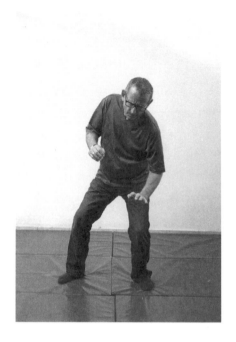

● EXERCISE

Put on some upbeat music of a big band or even a soul or disco group with a good rhythm.

The goal here is not to conduct them or dance to them – you're going to be part of them. Think of joining

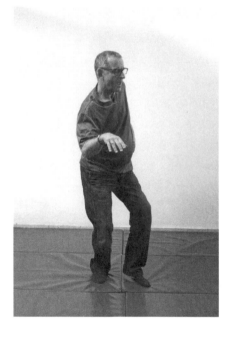

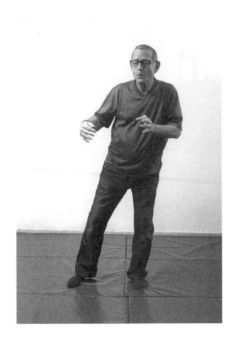

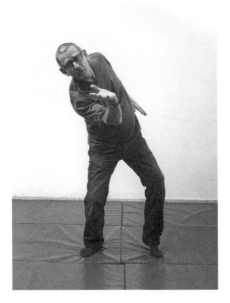

the best musicians in the world. They play and are paid well for it because that's what they know how to do. If you disturb them by not keeping the rhythm or playing bad notes, then you can't be part of them. *You have to make yourself part of them!*

You are now a musician and your instrument is your body. You can't imagine how great this feels. It doesn't matter if you play an instrument in real life. Because this *is* real life now.

A professional musician will give it his all, whether he is playing before 20 people in a jazz club or in front of a sold-out audience at Carnegie Hall. It's the same with a drummer, piano player, sax man, or bass player. And it's the same with a body player.

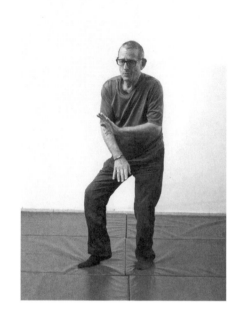

Enter into it and become the music. Feel the abdomen begin to go up and down, feel the shoulders become unstuck and move rhythmically. Why? Because you can't interrupt the music, you have to be the music. Your fellow musicians are counting on you, and if you screw up, the whole song is ruined.

When the trumpet or sax players go into a solo with lots of feeling, use your hands and play it. You'll make movements that you never imagined you could. It doesn't matter how silly you may look or how embarrassed you may be – forget about the outside world and become one with the instruments and your body.

Don't let your mind disturb you, let your mind become one with your body. Let your body lead you through movement, rhythm, and feelings.

Become the piano player and become the keyboard as the keys are being played. It will create new rhythms in your body you didn't realize that you had, or thought that were long lost.

Become the steady rhythms of the bass and the drums, and feel the solid sense of repetition and movement.

By the end of the song, besides feeling great, you'll discover that those musical rhythms that you just spent five or 10 minutes creating have become inscribed in you as strongly as the chaos of the Parkinson's. Your body wash has taken over.

If you still have energy – and you will – pick a different song with other instruments and rhythms and repeat the exercise. Your career as a body musician is in full swing.

When you become a trumpet player or a bass player in the body wash, you can also do it when you're not in the exercise. You can walk differently because you can say, "I'm a trumpet player, I'm a bass player... I'm a body player."

ALEX'S ENCOURAGEMENT

You can't play bad, you can only play good, and better. When you're a body player, you can play everywhere, even when there is no music. The music is in your head and 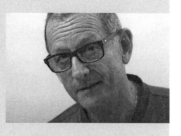 in your body – you can see it and hear it clearly as you go about your daily activities. And that's when you really start to see the results.

THOUGHT FOR THE DAY

Yesterday was terrible, but I'm not going to stay in yesterday – Today, I'm going to change it.

WHY IT WORKS

All life is a matter of balance, of being in the middle rhythmically, biochemically, and movement-wise. Some people call it the yin and yang of body and soul. It's our home base, our sense of physical and spiritual well-being. Knowing our middle state is one of the secrets of life.

EXERCISE 8: *Putting It All Together*

WHY THIS IS IMPORTANT

In the previous exercises, you've learned how to regain control of your breathing, your rhythm, and your movements. You've turned into conductors – using music, singers, and songs to free up your chest cavity, diaphragm, shoulders, legs, facial expressions, and hands.

You massaged yourselves internally by moving with abandon and freedom. In the process you've become unfrozen, you're no longer stiff, you've reduced your tremors, and you've increased your repertoire of movements beyond what you thought possible.

Now it's time to put it all together by realizing that music is life and that life is music. Through combining all of the exercises into one glorious and spontaneous dance of movement, you are learning to move from one situation to another and adapt your movements accordingly. It has huge implications for your daily life. Through these movements, you will be able to dance through life and all the challenges that face you.

The unexpected will no longer be frightening, but just another phase that you can pass through with grace and confidence.

● *EXERCISE*

In this exercise, you are your own teacher – you will feel the music and its rhythm and follow with improvisation and spontaneity.

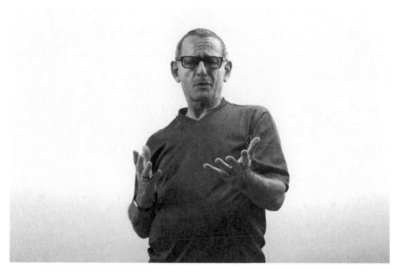

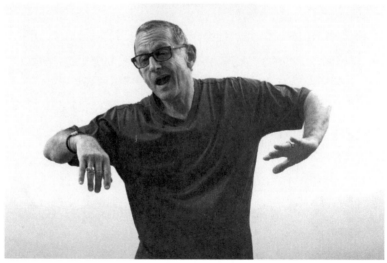

Choose music that provides you with headlines that take you through a story that has a beginning and end. If you become aware of your forms and movements and feel your facial and body forms, then you are in a position to be able to change them. Through music, rhythm,

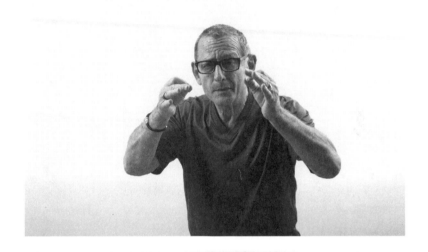

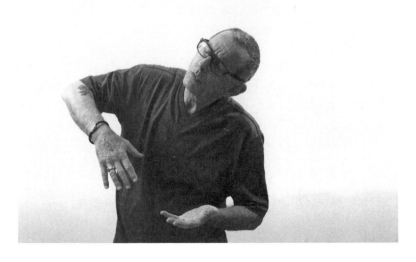

and movement, you can get in touch with your body and your feelings.

I have my own personal exercise that takes me on an emotion-filled excursion of expression and acting. My first headline is the soothing sounds of "Sentimental Journey."

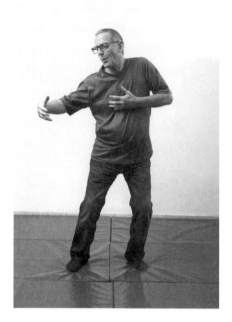

As the music plays, enter the song, feel the rhythm, and begin to move according to the emotions it's transmitting. Be expressive and throw your whole body into it with an internal body massage. Take the rhythm of this melancholy sentimental journey and express it through your body.

Remember to change your facial expression, using your entire arsenal: eyebrows, mouth, teeth, forehead, jaw, and even your nose. See how the face changes, the mouth opens and closes, the eyes go up and down. Work with the feelings and change the expression – be different! Be aware of the difference.

The next song picks up the pace and provides a different headline. With the more upbeat rhythm of

"Mack the Knife" by Bobby Darin, continue changing your facial expressions and enter inside the singer and the song with your body language. Improvise and activate your feelings! Give expression to the singer by imitating his cadence, rhythm, and breathing.

The swagger and big band sound will fill you with confidence and a sense of wellness. Embrace that confidence, express it with your hands, your shoulders, and your legs. Your repertoire of movements, which has been reduced by Parkinson's, has suddenly been incredibly increased!

If you find yourself getting too worked up and overstimulated, you can always return to the first song and slow things down. Or you can dance your movements slower even though the rhythm is faster. Remember, this is your exercise however you decide to build it.

Feel where you're stuck, feel your habit, and then feel the singer. How does he sing? How does he relate to his feelings? Let go, let your face open up.

You will notice that your breathing may become different, and you might begin to experience more tremors. That's very good! You've loosened up – don't stop!

You will become entrained to a new rhythm and new way of breathing. And you'll wonder where your tremors are.

The last headline is Paul Anka's version of Jon Bon Jovi's "It's My Life." What a lesson that is for us — *"It's my life and it's now or never"* and *"I just want to live while I'm alive."* Continue acting, imitating the singer with your facial expressions and moving your body into new forms. Meditate with the music in a free-form celebration.

Pay attention and you'll discover that you just learned something valuable through music: "It's my life and I'm not going to live forever." You experienced that headline and you're doing something about it that will enable you to live that life to its fullest.

Through these three headlines, you passed through movement massage, acting and facial expression, body language and breathing exercises with the singers. You went from home base rhythm to stimulated rhythm to back again.

You created a framework in which to feel good, one that can be changed each time, depending on the situation, your mood, and how you feel.

You learned to stop the thinking and enter your body, its language, its forms, and its feelings. You learned to express feelings that opened up your chest cavity, lungs, and digestive system. You just took your medication — a pill of rhythm, of music, and of feeling.

ALEX'S ENCOURAGEMENT

We act what we are
thinking and feeling.
Until now, we haven't
been aware that we're
acting out fear, acting our
survival syndrome, acting
Parkinson's. That script is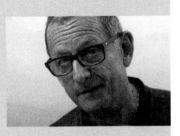
old – it's the past. We now have a new act – an act
of confidence, support, health, and happiness.

From now on, put on that act – make the facial
expressions, hand gestures, and body forms
of a healthy person. Instead of losing it, we are
using it – and our facial vocabulary will expand
and expand!

Parkinson's will no longer know where to be!

THOUGHT FOR THE DAY

Once you have proven that you can conduct, move
your hands, change your facial expressions and
body forms, the question arises: Why don't you do
it all the time? You've broken free from the spirit of
Parkinson's so don't tell me you can't do it. Don't
go back to your old habits.

WHY IT WORKS

When our breathing, body forms, and our eyes enter into a healthier entrainment, our autonomic nervous system works better and positively affects our dopamine, serotonin, and GABA neurotransmitters, bringing us to a balanced state.

Then the whole body tries to be in entrainment. We feel balanced, there is less chaos.

When are we in movement and rhythmic chaos? When those body movements and rhythms are not balanced. We're imbalanced when our breathing, eyes, and body forms are not in a balanced entrainment.

Once the body is in entrainment – for being diseased or healthy – that's the way the body acts. If we're in entrainment for being sick, then our survival syndrome and our body forms are working together to that end. That's exactly what we don't want.

EXERCISE 9: How to Sleep – An Excursion to Your Body

WHY THIS IS IMPORTANT

To sleep is an art – but you don't have to sleep in order to sleep.

Parkinson's patients say that they're tired during the day, and at night they're awake. You may wake up every night at three a.m. and start to worry. Your mind starts to work overtime and starts to churn out the endless barrage of scripts.

"Wow, I can't sleep. What am I going to do?" You start to eat, you watch TV, but most of all, you think and you worry. And it becomes chronic.

Lack of sleep is one of the Parkinson's patient's most debilitating symptoms. It can cause both psychological and physiological damage by taking you out of your alpha state and by irritating and amplifying all of the physical problems you are facing.

But even if you don't sleep, you can sleep. You can utilize your awake time by connecting with your body.

You can have a session with your psychotherapist, meaning simply sitting and being aware that your body is speaking with your mind.

The body will tell you: I feel very tense, I don't have the right movement in my abdomen, I'm tight in my chest, my breathing and heartbeat are not in entrainment. I even feel sad.

There's a conversation going on and you're now in treatment with your psychotherapist – yourself. And you're the best psychotherapist that there could ever be.

Generally when you go to a therapist, you go with your mind, not your body. But when the mind hears the body, it enables a change to take place. There's movement. You'll feel it in your abdomen and in your heart.

Everything will become clearer because you spoke with yourself and your body.

● *EXERCISE*

We're going on an excursion to the body.

Sit in a relaxed position, close your eyes, and breathe rhythmically through your mouth.

Feel how the breath enters your abdomen. It's expanding and contracting.

Breathe to the maximum capacity of your lungs until you feel your abdomen is full, and exhale slowly.

Feel it – be there. Don't think about it, just feel what's going on there.

Repeat the deep breathing a few times and enter a rhythm.

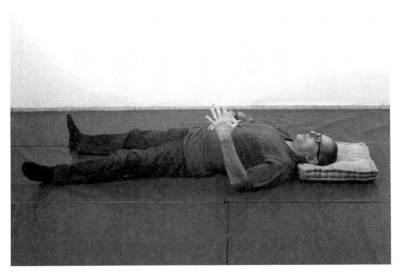

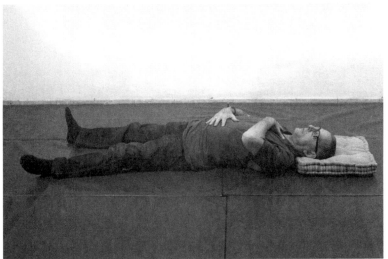

Now keep doing it but focus on your chest cavity
– enter into it. Feel movement there. Something is
happening but don't think about it. Keep your eyes
closed and remain there.

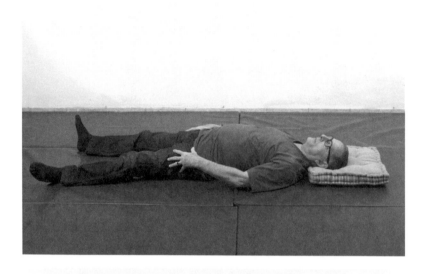

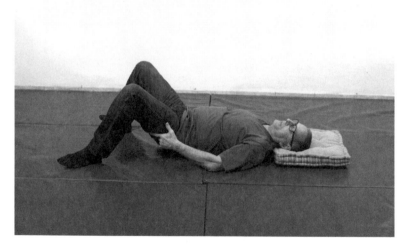

Feel how your abdomen and chest cavities are working together and both moving. Remember the springs? They are contracting and expanding and returning to their original form, not the Parkinson's form.

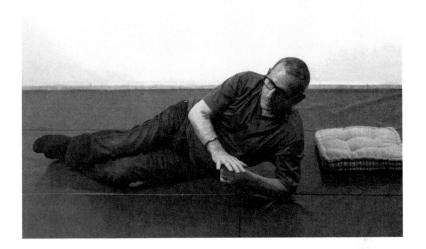

Now, focus on the area between your abdomen and chest. Feel your diaphragm, and in the middle of the diaphragm, you'll feel your heart.

Try to feel the heart pumping. Concentrate on the heartbeat and breathe into it. You'll feel exactly where your abdomen and chest cavities are divided. Breathe...

The wordless conversation taking place with your body is as good as a deep, refreshing sleep. You're in your interval zone, your alpha state. There is no story from the past or the future in your eyes. Concentrate on them, and they will tell a story that is totally in the present.

Feel your mouth. See how it's relaxed, no longer tense and waiting for the next twinge of pain to come.

Continue your rhythmic breathing – feel your abdomen, chest, heartbeat, eyes, mouth, and facial expression.

You're in communion with your body. Don't think. Just feel and sleep.

Enjoy. It's a good feeling. It's a great calming exercise. Remain there, entwined with your body in harmony and a sense of well-being.

Open your eyes slowly. How do you feel?

There should be a sense of contentment, tranquility, and even though you weren't asleep in the traditional sense, a feeling of being rested.

Then notice something — where is your Parkinson's? It's not there like it was before. It's something different.

Get up and you'll be amazed at how wonderful you feel. Just by concentrating on the basic areas of your body, communicating with them and blocking out the scripts from your mind, you were able to return to your alpha state and get in contact with yourself.

Your body told you what it was feeling and you responded, like any good psychotherapist would, with love and understanding. By letting go of the mind and focusing on the body, the anxiety and stress over not sleeping has melted away.

ALEX'S ENCOURAGEMENT

We all have to unlearn
the process of constantly
thinking and creating
stories in our mind. This is
vital for everyone, not just
people with Parkinson's.

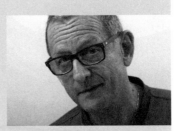

Stop the anxiety and
the scripts now! Enter the interval zone, your
home base, and feel good. That's all. Sleep will
then come.

THOUGHT FOR THE DAY

Change your inner dialogue and be aware of the
words you use. Use happier and healthy language
– words are very powerful and energizing.

EXERCISE 10: Beginners

If your situation is severe, or if you want to tentatively test out the various forms of movement exercises that are available, then use this as a beginners' guide that can help ease you into the world of movement.

All of these beginner exercises are designed to build awareness of your body systems, your feelings, and the movements within your body. They help to increase your movement span and decrease the sense of being frozen or stuck.

MOVEMENT IS LIFE… NO MOVEMENT IS DEATH!

● EXERCISE A

Put on relaxing background music, not too rhythmic or raucous – pop standards with strings and lots of emotion will work well. Slow rhythms are for soothing, relaxing, and healing emotional movements.

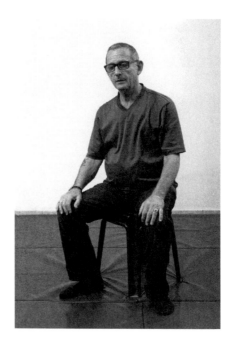

Sit comfortably with your feet apart and hands on knees. It can be on a chair or

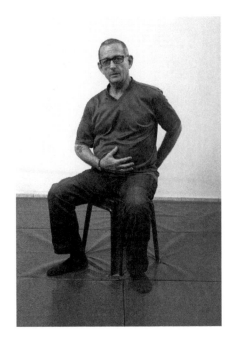

on the floor if that is comfortable. Your eyes can be open or closed.

It is very important to breathe through your mouth and forcefully exhale, because you speak, sing, and train physically by exhaling rhythmically.

Exhale rhythmically in most of the movements you do: writing, wearing clothes, reading, expressing yourself, and doing physical work.

The more you exhale, the better you will inhale!

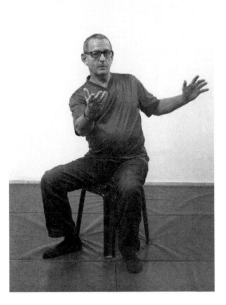

Listen to the music. Don't think, just listen. Breathe in harmony with the singer or instrument. Become one with the music, breathe it and feel it, and slowly start to move with the music.

Express your feelings through your face and hands – move them and express yourself – change your body language and enter it! Don't stay stuck!

You're becoming one with the music – don't think about it, feel it!

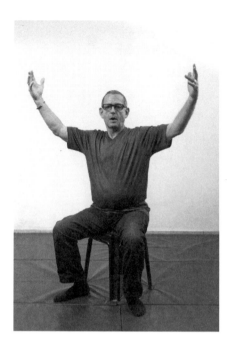

● *EXERCISE B*

Repeat Exercise A while standing. See how much more movement there is.

● *EXERCISE C*

Self-Massage

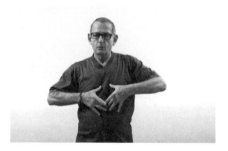

Close your eyes while standing and let the music move through your body and all of its systems. Start with your feet and knees and move up through your thighs, pelvis, and vertebrae into your shoulders, elbows, and hands.

Feel the slow, melodic rhythmic movements of the music within your body. Add your neck and your facial expressions. All of your body is loosening up and moving differently.

● *EXERCISE D*

Building on Exercise C, begin to move even more by imitating and becoming the singer of the song. Breathe the way he sings, imitate his body language and his emotions. Sing if you want, or lip-synch if it's more comfortable.

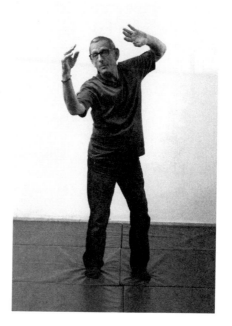

Then become a conductor and conduct the band and the singer, leading them through the song.

● *EXERCISE E*

Pretend that you're swimming and swim according to the rhythm of the music. Breathe and move according to the swimming style.

EXERCISE 11: Intermediate

You are now up on your feet and ready to start moving faster. Medium rhythms are for body movement – rhythm entrainment, and these exercises start you on the way to entrain your movement and rhythm in your body that has become used to the chaotic and irregular rhythmic movements of Parkinson's.

● EXERCISE A

Put on a midtempo song, whether it be a samba or a rhythmic pop song.

Start to move with the rhythm and concentrate on your feet. When you are comfortable with that, begin to breathe rhythmically with the movement of your feet.

When that's going well, start to swing your hands in coordination with your feet and breathing. Continue moving and synchronize your hand and body movements with your feet and rhythmic breathing.

You'll discover that it's not only lots of fun, but very effective. It helps to build up the "rhythm" within your body that has been short-circuited by the Parkinson's, and it gives you a good workout.

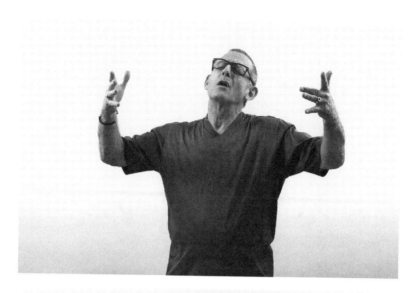

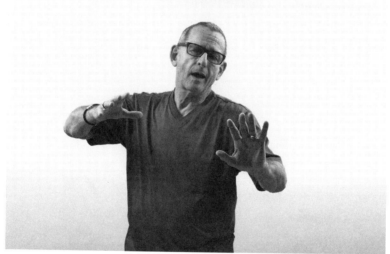

● *EXERCISE B*

Change the music to something even faster and more dynamic – like upbeat Latin music or disco. Fast-paced music is for energetically stimulating the body's rhythmic movements.

Begin a repeat of Exercise A and when you get into a good rhythm, start to do some improvising in an attempt to change your body forms. Try to be as light, easy, and springy as possible. Focus on different parts of your body and get them to move to the music.

These two exercises will provide you with a very effective inventory of combinations of movement and fill you with rhythm and energy. You'll be so energized that you'll forget to be stuck and frozen.

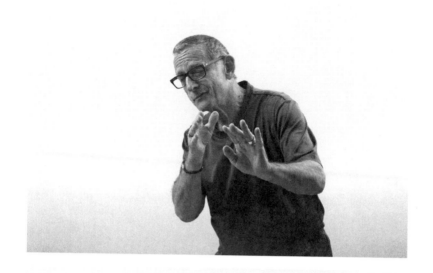

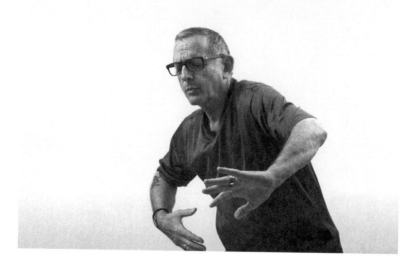

EXERCISE 12: Advanced

Once you are comfortable with the active energy of the music and have begun to regain your rhythm and found entrainment between your body movements and your breathing and rhythm, you can move on to advanced exercises that will take you to a new plateau.

● *EXERCISE A*

We're still using the fast-paced songs of disco or Latin. Listen to the music and warm up with Exercise 2. When you're ready, try to become one with the rhythm section. It's a steady beat and, using your upper hands, waist, and abdomen, foot movements and techniques – moving to the side and to the back – you become the dancer of the rhythm section.

It's fun, athletic, and effective.

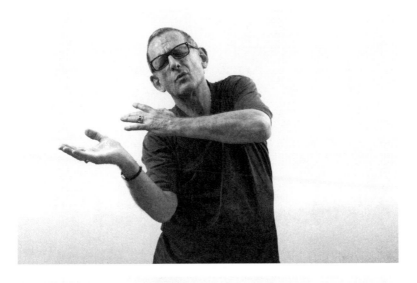

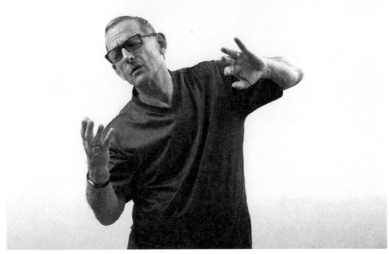

● *EXERCISE B*

This is where free dancing, the art of movement, body language, acting, and improvisation come together. It's all a matter of what the body wants when you embark on the exercise.

There is no "thinking" in this exercise, just feeling and movement.

Put on any free, expressive music, whether it be classical or modern ballet accompaniment.

And just let go and see where the music takes you. Use your newly discovered movement potential and inventory of movement to go where you haven't gone before.

That inventory will help you make big changes in your life.

Repeat all of the exercises as often as you can or need to. There is no fast rule, but the more you practice and master them, the more they will become inscribed in your body and mind. And that means the more it will take hold even when you're not on the exercise mat.

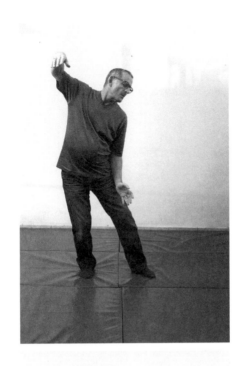

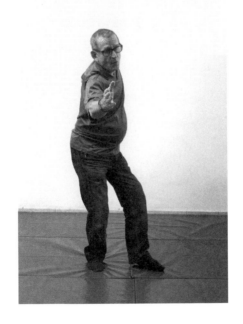

EXERCISE 13: Finishing Up

For all exercises: Lie on your back and relax. Stop thinking and let the clutter in your mind clear out. Release every part of your body – feel your different body parts.

Breathe into your abdominal cavity and feel the movements within your abdomen. Remember to breathe with your mouth open and concentrate on exhaling.

Continue to breathe into your abdomen and fill your chest cavity, feel the movements.

Concentrate on your heartbeat and breathe into it rhythmically until your breathing and heartbeat become one.

Release the tenseness in your face. Feel your facial expressions. Experience the power of "feeling" and stop thinking.

Feel your body… don't think!!

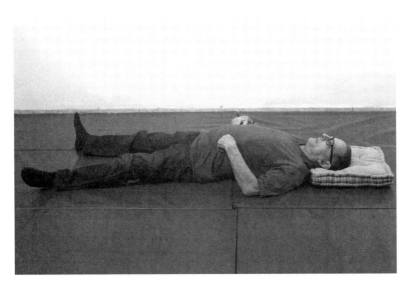

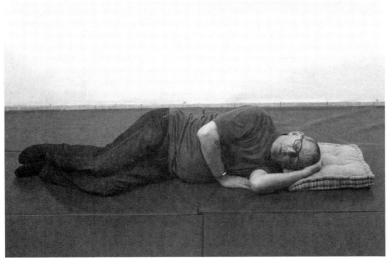

ALEX'S ENCOURAGEMENT

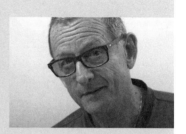

If you can stop thinking while you exercise and forget about your Parkinson's, you can stop thinking when you go to the movies, when you read a book, or when you're in a restaurant. By establishing a rhythm for yourself, you can do anything. By not thinking, you can do anything. Be in the present.

THOUGHT FOR THE DAY

All of a sudden you'll see you breathe differently. Then you can guide yourself to the healthy destination of where you want to be.

LOSING MY WALKER

by DORIS CORONEL

I am 52 years old and was diagnosed with Parkinson's disease about nine years ago.

When the neurologist who diagnosed me made sure that I understood that "Parkinson's is a progressive, degenerative neurological condition that only gets worst with time, and there is no cure for it," I decided to empower myself and learn as much as I could about this condition.

I clearly remember deciding that I was not going to sit and cry about it, but instead, I was going to see it as a "challenge." Parkinson's was not going to conquer me. Over the next five years, I kept to my routines without any major problems; I worked, exercised, walked, and ran. I took enough medication to have a therapeutic effect with minimal side effects. I did not feel the need to share my condition with my colleagues and not even with my extended family.

The last three years have been a different story. My ability to walk became more impaired, and I started shuffling a great deal. I was very tired during the day, and I became self-conscious about my looks. My writing became smaller, almost illegible, and my posture deteriorated even more.

But the worst thing was that in this process, I was also losing my self-confidence. Because I was so afraid of falling, I started isolating myself, turning down invitations from my friends to go out, and emphasizing my shortcomings and my limitations, instead of my strengths.

Unconsciously, I was impairing myself more than I really was, by "assuming" that because I had Parkinson's, I would not be able to do certain things. Parkinson's took over my life. By now, I was walking with a cane, with which I developed a "love/hate" relationship.

I stopped walking the dog, I stopped riding my bike, I stopped going to the gym, I even missed work events with large groups of people, like conferences and workshops. Life works in unexpected ways. Sometimes, when we think that all the doors are closing on us, a window opens and we see the sunshine again. This happened to me recently. My brother-in-law sent me an article from an Israeli magazine about a former martial instructor who was doing innovative work with Parkinson's patients called Gyro-Kinetics.

After having tried almost all Parkinson's medications with negative side effects, after trying unconventional approaches such as acupuncture, touch for health, lifeline techniques, tai chi, and osteopathic remedies without long-lasting results, I felt more than ready to listen to what my gut feeling had to say. My instinct was touched by the philosophy behind the Gyro-Kinetics approach, which simply put was "to help move from being a professional Parkinson's patient to being a healthy person with Parkinson's."

A few weeks later, I arrived in Israel, using a walker, since the cane was no longer doing the job. I met Alex Kerten and his staff and he explained how the program worked.

After struggling for the previous three years with doctors, medications, and different opinions, it's difficult to explain with words the impact that this ten-day, two-and-a-half-to-three-hours-a-day program had on me. The first thing that I regained was my self-confidence; and the first thing I lost, after three days, was my walker.

In essence, the key to the program is to act like we don't have Parkinson's so the PD gets "confused" when the body acts in a different way than expected. To deprogram ourselves, we need to substitute our long-term memory with new long-term memory by changing our behavior.

This takes time and a lot of patience. But mostly, it takes a teacher willing to be there for his students, a teacher who is disciplined, consistent, reliable, honest, tough, and who never gives up. That teacher is Alex Kerten. He doesn't treat his students with kid gloves or sugarcoat the treatment but instead delivers a clear and conscious message. He does not allow his clients to be mediocre; he wants them to use all their potential, just as he does.

Alex's program showed me that there is hope, that there are possibilities to improve, and techniques to use.

In order to benefit from his program, you need to be willing to try something very different and be able to tolerate frustration. It will pay off.

SECTION 3

KEEP GOING!

Chapter 16

Where Does Medication Fit In?

You've gone to the doctor because you've been experiencing the symptoms of Parkinson's, and he tells you something like this: "OK, I'm going to prescribe some medication for you — one is to stimulate your dopamine to spark your nervous system and the other is to stimulate your serotonin to keep you calm. Let's meet again in a half year."

During that six-month period, you find yourself becoming depressed, with no energy. When you go back, the doctor says, "All right, let's make some adjustments to try and straighten it out" and he may prescribe more or different medication.

It's a rare instance when he would stop and say, "Why do you look like that in your eyes? Look at your chest, your breathing, your tremors. You're looking very Parkinsonian."

Instead, he may send you to a respiratory specialist or to an eye doctor to work on those specific issues. They may suggest things they don't even understand, like "go do tai chi, walk more, take some movement classes."

Is there a doctor who will look you in the eye and say, "What is wrong here is your behavior patterns. *You have to change your behavior.*"?

But that is precisely what you must do, and if you've read this far, you know how to do that. The moment the actor understands that he is responsible for the role and he is not controlled by the scenario given to him, something very interesting takes place.

Let's say you go to a doctor and he gives you the standard Parkinson's diagnosis, recommending medication to slow down the deterioration.

However, it soon becomes clear that medication may be able to help you with symptom A while causing new symptoms B and C. Another medication solves C but brings with it other side effects. In many cases, the medical cocktail prescribed may become a bigger problem than your PD itself!

When you're presented with the Parkinson's scenario, you have a choice. You can decide to follow the medical advice and sign up to be a professional Parkinson's patient. Or you can thank the doctor and tell him you'll think about what he said. You have the right to decide what is best for your life — and you definitely have the right to search for a second opinion.

Then, before you enter the spirit of Parkinson's with a regimen of medication, side effects, and deterioration, you can decide to enter a zone where you have the opportunity to neutralize Parkinson's by listening to your body and communicating and interacting with your body/mind potential.

This will enable you to improve the way your body reacts to Parkinson's. Then, when you return to the doctor in a better state of health and balance and in a good relationship with yourself, he will be able to prescribe less medication that will have better effects.

Parkinsonism

When you go back to the doctor in six months in better mind/body interaction, he might say, "I see some signs of Parkinsonism, but not PD." That's a big difference.

As we learned earlier, Parkinsonism is stage one of Parkinson's disease. Parkinsonism means that you have Parkinson's, but it's not professional Parkinson's. You have some symptoms but it doesn't have to develop or get worse, and your condition doesn't have to deteriorate.

You can live with it, and sometimes you can even say "thank you" to Parkinson's because it brought you closer to your body and gave you a sense of proportion. You're able to regularly tell yourself, "OK, let's stay balanced, don't wear myself out, don't burn out."

I've seen it happen dozens of times, and the medical establishment doesn't understand it. "How can it be that you feel better now than when you first came in?"

The answer is that we began to listen to our body. The body began to tell the mind that the Parkinson's script was wrong for him and when they began to work together, the mind provided a new script called *being healthy*.

Medication

The biggest obstacle to fighting Parkinson's is the medication – the complicated cocktails of drugs that can cause side effects we're not even aware of. We end up becoming a slave to those side effects and their own scenarios as much as we have to our Parkinson's symptoms.

Take medication to help uplift you, but remember that it's your responsibility to feel good.

So first of all try to feel good. And when you feel good, your pharmacology works better. Then you can decide how to take medication.

By changing your own pharmacology, by conducting, moving, and getting out of the spirit of Parkinson's, your levels of the neurotransmitters dopamine and serotonin begin to change, and they can affect your GABA, which inspires your body rhythms.

Patients who came to me could hardly move at the beginning. But I was able to change their rhythm and their state of mind. And all of a sudden, their pharmacology changed – and this is the secret power of the brain. Don't limit it, give it the potential to expand. Let your brain be jazzy and improvise – don't limit it with classic words and classic medication. The brain knows how to improvise and make combinations and to jam – and the result is you suddenly have a better balance among dopamine, GABA, and serotonin. Once you give the brain and the body the ability to work together and systematically bring them to a new home base, miracles take place.

Now, when you go to the doctor, the medication prescribed based on the symptoms will be a much lower level and can greatly help you instead of being debilitating and leading to harmful side effects.

Making Medication Count

Because the digestive system of a Parkinson's patient is already acting according to the scenario of the future, there might be ongoing constipation. This can have a drastic effect on the medicine that the patient is taking — 50% of the medication goes down the toilet and only 50% to the brain. It's very important that your digestive system is working correctly while taking medication.

So if you're able to change the script and leave your anxiety-ridden state for the present, your digestive system should work fine, the medication will be more effective, and you will be able to lower the dosage to the minimum.

By living in the present, your autonomic nervous system acts according to the present. If you can stay there, it creates the suitable environment for your Parkinson's to also change forms. And your need for high dosages of medications may also change for the better.

No pharmacy can equal our own pharmacology!

Chapter 17

The Role of Music

I lost myself in a familiar song
I closed my eyes and I slipped away
— Boston (*More Than a Feeling*)

Music is life. Music is the expression of all the experiences we have in our lives. The way we speak, from the way we say "good morning" to the way we say "good night," is colored by the tone, cadence, and rhythm we create.

We can reveal so much about ourselves and our mood by the way we speak. A jovial operatic "GOOD MORNING" gives such a different message from a monotone, perfunctory "G'morning… ."

And the way we greet someone also has a tremendous impact on the person on the receiving end. If our boss offers us that bright, cheerful, and musical greeting, we're going to feel differently (much better) than if he gives us that nonmusical mumbling nod.

Everything in our daily life has music and rhythm in it. We hear it in a horse's hooves, in birds, the rustle of trees — it's all around us. If we accept the fact that music isn't only the songs we hear on the radio but a way of life, then our ears and minds will realize that music is everywhere.

It's the same with our bodies and movement. The way we eat, breathe, brush our teeth, walk, and run are all based on the rhythm of our internal music.

I mentioned when I talked about my life story that I was once a professional musician, performing with some of the biggest international stars who visited Israel in the 1960s. As I moved on to other phases of my life, I stopped playing an instrument for over 20 years. When I returned to it, I realized something: music has an effect on my subconscious.

Music has its own scripts and stories that can significantly stimulate our brain with its own stories and stimulate our body rhythmically. If we can translate music to motor movements, then we can create new facts.

By using music and the art of movement, people who are limited in using their hands or can't move certain body parts or have frozen faces can suddenly conduct and make facial expressions. And if we can train ourselves to behave rhythmically in an automatic fashion, then it will lead to some incredible changes in our lives.

Patients come to me and they don't realize that there is music in their voice, there is rhythm in their voice, and that they still have their own facial expressions. It is just being masked by the Parkinson's.

Through music and exercises involving conducting, the art of movement through free dancing, and internal massage, we are going to regain our movement inventory that has been strangled by Parkinson's. We are going to speak with our body, change our facial expression, and breathe together with the singer and band. And by using these techniques, we are going to learn something we already knew: how to look healthy and to be healthy.

When we put on music with a strong rhythm – like a Sousa marching band anthem – we immediately begin to find our internal rhythm and begin to gain the confidence of a Parkinson's warrior. We let the music and its rhythm become our teacher, instructing us how to move and how to breathe.

We begin to move differently than we do in our daily routine, where we have become used to a Parkinson's way of movement. We're changing how we move because of the rhythm of the music.

Music is the strongest medication available to us. It enters into us rhythmically, harmony-wise, and subject-wise. We become part of music's many stories, which allows us to neutralize our own story.

Whenever we hear music, it is informed by our past – that's why it has such a strong effect on us. Hearing a song can immediately bring us back to a certain moment in our life and dredge up strong feelings.

At the same time, music helps us become one with our body. As we listen to the music, move to the music, and breathe to the music, our rhythm and our body shapes undergo miraculous changes.

What Kind of Music, What Kind of Mood?

If we want to feel balanced, in our alpha state, we should put on music with a steady but medium rhythm – no upbeat rock or disco. Some good midtempo pop is fine – or if you prefer classical, there's Tchaikovsky or Bach.

If we want to get stimulated and get our body moving, try some Latin music, bossa nova, or samba. It will give a feeling of elevation. For classical, try some of the more explosive pieces by Stravinsky or Rachmaninoff.

When we want to enter our body and conduct inwardly, we need to take a slow, soothing rhythm – "Put Your Head on My Shoulders" or "You Are the Sunshine of My Life" or another lush classic love song.

Ultimately, the goal of music is bring us to our home base, where we feel like we're in an alpha state of balance, with our rhythm and our heartbeat working in entrainment, in coordination.

However, as we have learned is the case with many Parkinson's sufferers, the excited beta rhythm is their home base. We're going to do a reset – bringing our home base back to alpha. When we do a reset by fasting and cleansing our body, our body will tell us what it wants to eat. Likewise, with music, our body will tell us what it wants to hear.

So ask your body, "What do you want?" And then do what it says.

Let the song, singer, and musicians be your teacher.

Chapter 18

The Role of the Spouse/ Caregiver

The impact of Parkinson's isn't felt only by the person with the disease. The symptoms affect everyone he or she comes in contact with – the closer you are to a Parkinson's patient, the greater effect it will have on your life.

That means that a Parkinson's patient's spouse or life partner – who invariably becomes the primary caregiver for their loved one – is in the front lines of the battle against the disease. And that can be very problematic if not handled correctly.

According to the National Parkinson's Foundation, caregiver stress comes part and parcel of providing for someone with a long-developing chronic illness such as PD. "Compassion fatigue" and even exhaustion can take a toll on both physical and emotional health.

The foundation's website provides a long list of symptoms that caregivers begin to experience that worsen as the disease progresses, including:

- An ongoing tendency to ignore or postpone taking care of one's own health needs.

- Growing feelings of isolation, as in, "Nobody knows or understands what is really going on with us."
- Feelings of anxiety, uncertainty about the future, a "waiting for the other shoe to drop" crisis. This could trigger verbal or even physical abuse of the care recipient.
- Feelings of anger at the care recipient or situation, often followed by guilt.

After working with hundreds of patients and wives or husbands who turn into primary caregivers, I've developed some tips that will help the caregiver cope with their new situation. In addition to assisting their partner in the most positive way, these tips will enable them to continue their pre-Parkinson's lives as closely as possible.

Carry On Your Life

The caregiver needs to realize and internalize the idea that the most important part of their work is to provide a normal life routine despite the changing circumstances.

This means remembering how to feel good, feel happy, and feel social – don't fall into the trap of taking on the script of Parkinsonism. Don't take on the responsibility of your partner's Parkinson's, otherwise you might become even more afflicted than your partner!

Don't make plans taking Parkinson's into consideration. "We can't go to our weekly bridge game anymore; we can't go out to the movies and be around all those people." That way of thinking is wrong — because all of a sudden the script becomes Parkinson's for the both of you.

Even if you as a couple didn't generally go out much before the Parkinson's, it's more important now that you deliberately start to go out. Don't sequester yourselves in your home!

You may find yourself increasingly doing all of your partner's work for him — cutting the food on his plate, opening his button, closing his belt, helping, helping, helping! It becomes a chronic automatic reaction.

As caregiver, you must always be aware that your priority needs to be to stay healthy yourself and to be as happy as possible. In order to do this, you should be consulting with your partner. Discuss issues together like "How can we continue to live happily? How can we continue to lead our lives in a positive and social way?"

It's important to create an atmosphere for a healthy person and not for a sick, diseased person. That way, the script that you both follow will be more likely to be based on feelings of health and not sickness.

Exercising with Your Partner

Doing the exercises in this book jointly with your Parkinson's partner can be a great experience. The movement through conducting and dancing is beneficial for you, too. I have couples who not only enjoy themselves, but through the art of movement, they've become even closer to each other. They've begun to listen to each other, and communication has become better.

I would recommend it as long as you can avoid analyzing, judging, or criticizing. Be open-minded and avoid exerting control over your "weaker" partner. Saying "Do it this way," "Why are you moving like that?" or "You're doing it wrong" will have the opposite effect and drive the two of you apart. And your partner will stop listening to you.

So stop analyzing and leading, and enjoy yourselves together.

Be Supportive

Don't judge or criticize to the extreme — nurture and encourage without babying. If you constantly criticize your partner that he's not doing enough and letting the Parkinson's get the better of him, he's going to phase you out and stop listening.

Speak to him like the body and mind are supposed to speak. When he is working on the exercises and the breathing techniques, then be like the body speaking to him: "How can I help you? I see that you are trying so hard. My dear, it's beautiful what you are accomplishing."

And if you see that he's not trying so hard, be firm and remind him that it's his responsibility. "I'm not going to take on that role for you. If you don't work hard, then I'm not going to take your disease upon myself."

Because if that scenario does become a reality and the caregiver takes on more and more responsibility as the patient slowly gives up the battle, then you'll both start down a long, slippery slope. Your partner will see that you are doing the work so he won't have to. And all of a sudden, he will stop doing things, stop going out, and you'll have to push him more and more.

By taking away the responsibility of the patient for his own actions, it enables him to remain in his past behavior. The end result is that he will go one way, and his partner/caregiver will go the other way. And they may never meet up again, resulting in heartache and tension that only exacerbates the already challenging situation.

Ultimately, both the Parkinson's patient and the caregiver have their own responsibilities. It's the PD sufferer's responsibility to ensure that his spouse or partner has the option to continue to be happy. And it's the caregiver's responsibility to ensure the continuity of life as usual.

The most dangerous thing is if the caregiver starts thinking along the lines of, "Well, he's got Parkinson's. It will be too difficult or embarrassing to go out. We'll stay home."

Because all of a sudden, the caregiver turns into the partner's disease even more than the Parkinson's is.

Don't let it happen!

Helpful Tips

Tremors

There are situations when tremors do not occur consistently: they attack, suddenly. We know that fatigue and stress can contribute to tremors and trembling, which leads to muscle fatigue and vice versa.

- Focus on your breathing, loosen your hands and shoulder muscles, and be aware of your facial expressions.

- Transform the tremors into voluntary movements: conduct, express yourself – but don't let the "broken" movements created by the trembling guide you. Transform them into flowing movements and don't forget to keep breathing rhythmically.

- Make exercise and physical activity part of your daily routine: yoga, Feldenkreis, dance, and the Gyro-Kinetic method. Get frequent massages, and rest occasionally. Listen to your body!

- Sometimes, if your tremors cannot be controlled, try this exercise. Stand with your legs apart and deliberately enter a trembling state with your whole body. Then cool down, and stop the deliberate tremors. You'll see that some of the uncontrollable tremors have also subsided.

Walking

The loss of equilibrium and incorrect posture make normal, healthy walking difficult. Small, fast steps placing your feet close together and keeping your heels or toes in the air may all cause the loss of equilibrium.

- Slow down, check your posture, sway from side to side with your legs apart, and focus on your breathing rhythms.

- When swaying from side to side, focus your glance a point or two ahead of you. When walking, keep a comfortable space between your legs (at least as wide as the pelvis), breathe rhythmically and march rhythmically ("left/right" or "forward march!").

- Raise your knees when walking. Use your posterior muscles instead of dragging your feet – this will prevent you from falling if you encounter an obstacle.

- Use your hands while walking and match their movements to your breathing rhythm.

- When turning around, use the same method: sway from leg to leg while raising your knees and start to turn around. Practice as often as possible.

Falling

Parkinson's affects the brain's equilibrium and coordination centers. The body's balance, which was previously an automatic function, becomes increasingly difficult and results in damaged posture and a tendency to fall.

- If you lose your balance, exhale as hard as you can and reach your hands forward to an object that can be held on to (or even an imaginary one). Alternatively, put your hands on your thighs. Your body will bend forward automatically and, generally, prevent the fall. If you do fall, this routine will prevent a more dangerous fall backward.

- If you sense that you are losing your equilibrium, try to plan your fall forward. Try to slow down your movements while falling, as if it was planned. Remember to exhale – this will support movement control.

Rigidity

Attempting to move while in an "off" or rigid situation can worsen the situation and result in a fall.

- When "frozen," don't attempt to walk. Sway from side to side and try to regain control of your breathing rhythm. Then look straight ahead, walking rhythmically in place. Choose a target and then walk toward it.

- Follow the same procedure if you're in an "off" position. Breathe rhythmically, be aware of your facial expressions, move your hands rhythmically as if you were a bird, or start conducting, or make any movement that could change your mood. Continue moving in place until you sense that you are in control of your situation, and then start walking forward.

Speech

Many people with Parkinson's have general speech difficulties, particularly when attempting clear or loud speech.

- Study the coordination between breathing and speech rhythms. Speak slowly, emphasize punctuation, pause between words, and use your hands to stress the point.

- Overstate punctuation and facial expressions – "act out" the words and sentences as if you were onstage and facing an audience.

- Repeat the same procedure when talking on the telephone.

- Address the audience, stare at them in the eyes, and try to get them to understand you. Remember that you are onstage.

- Accompany your speech with slow, rhythmic breaths – express the words while exhaling. Speak briefly, be concise and decisive. Simplify your intentions.

Lying to Standing

- Practice as often as you can, on a carpet, mattress, or floor.

- Imagine that you are an animal that walks on all fours.

- Make movements that are as varied as possible; crawl, roll over, and move forward and backward while feeling your physical potential.

- Fold your legs toward your abdomen; move them from side to side and then add the pelvis to the movement. Balance your body on your elbows and raise yourself to an all fours position. After practicing this routine on the floor, you arrive at the harder part – practicing the same routine from your bed.

Standing from Sitting Position

- Sit on the edge of a bed, put both feet on the floor, place your hands on the sides of your body, and bow the upper part of your body forward.

- Repeat the bow a few times while breathing rhythmically. Then bow, exhale, and push yourself forward to a standing position with your head leaning down and forward and raising your posterior upward and forward. When you do that, your head will raise itself automatically and you can then stand up.

- When your posterior is raised backward, your head will lean downward and your posture will be bent. When pushing your posterior forward, your body will straighten.

Listen to your body and be aware of its movement potential.

- Learn your body language — that's how it talks to you through feelings, rhythm, and movement.
- Stimulate the mind — build new neural connections. Visit new places, watch films, sing, dance, and challenge yourself.
- Be positive and enthusiastic. Remember that a healthy mood (psychological) has an effect on the hormonal secretions (biological), which has a direct effect on the body (physiological).

The goal of your treatment is to feel good and become a healthy person with Parkinson's. You can do it!

Conclusion: Making It Part of Your Life

"By my body's actions teach my mind."
— William Shakespeare

If I'm going to learn how to speak a new language, I could attempt it in one of two ways. I could go to a lesson for an hour, practice, then leave and go back to speaking English in my comfort zone. Then the next time I go to a lesson, I'll start all over again.

Or, I can immerse myself in the new language and make it a part of my life. I have to practice and have it enter my being 24 hours a day. It's the same with training ourselves to say goodbye to Parkinson's disease. If we want to do anything in life – speak French, get physically fit, change our habits – we have to prepare ourselves and start doing it! All the time!

Your body is an automatic expression of your habits. If you keep your habits and your Parkinsonian body forms, your Parkinson's will stay with you. You can change your body forms and your habits and your Parkinson's will also change.

In the previous chapters, you've learned how to reduce your percentage of Parkinson's. Listen to your body and discover what it's telling you. Remember, Parkinson's, pain, and fatigue are all information that you can use.

Use it to bring your mind and body together to work as a team so you can change the habits and the forms, and with time, reduce your percentage of Parkinson's.

Using New Movements

When I treat a person who was cervically injured and needs to learn how to walk again, I must teach him new movements. At first, he tries to imitate his old movements, but they will never come to him again. I teach him new movements and that's what he knows.

When the film *The King's Speech* came out with Colin Firth, people said, "Wow – it's amazing!" But for me, what the therapist did with him was so natural. If you can't do it one way, then do it a different way. If you stutter, then use tools to change the rhythm of your speech. If you have tremors or are stuck, then change your body's rhythm and your body forms.

If you go to see a play in a Parkinsonian state, you may get "stuck" trying to enter the theater. People will start to shout, "Hey, will you move?" and you may get even more stuck.

But if you have the capability to dance through the line, then you're no longer even in the theater in mind or body. You can go through dancing and improvise your movements because you learned from the art of movement and free dancing to go from one situation to another and adapt to the changing realities.

It's applicable whether you're going to a restaurant, having an argument with your spouse, or sitting with your doctor when he gets annoyed with you for expressing your point of view.

A New Inscription

You've learned to let your body know that you are listening to it and adopt the correct behavior. Whether you're conducting, breathing rhythmically, or dancing, you are not going to work on it, feel good, and then go back to Parkinson's. No way!

You're going to practice and use it as a powerful tool against Parkinson's. And believe me, it is very powerful.

Spending 30 or 40 minutes a day on these exercises will open you up to the realization and awareness of the need to bring this way of thinking into your life. It will be inscribed in your mind and your body. You'll begin to understand the metaphor of conducting your way through life, of free movement and dancing so you know how to move from one situation to another without getting stuck, and of internal massage so you realize how your body really behaves when treated properly.

You'll also internalize how important it is to respect your body and speak to it and understand what it is telling you. Our mind is always trying to translate what the body says. But they are speaking two different languages. The body speaks through feelings and body forms – the mind answers it through sentences. But when the mind and body understand each other, the whole world can change.

But by conducting and meditating on your different body systems – the abdominal cavity, the diaphragm – and on your breathing and rhythm, and feeling what is happening in your chest cavity, and how you're expressing yourself with your hands and your face, you will become aware of your body.

And then it becomes a state of mind. And state of mind equals the forms your body takes. "I'm in the body form of love, the form of jealousy. I'm in the form of Parkinson's. I'm in the form of being healthy!"

Understanding is psychology, behavior is physiology. Rely on your understanding, rely on your behavior and only then, your medication will become more effective.

These are the tools. Now make them part of your life.

Be aware of "feeing bad" and being stuck. Feel bad about feeling bad – IT'S OK! Feel bad about it until you make a new habit of feeling good.

It's very hard work, but the habit of "feeling good" contains tremendous power. Don't let "feeling bad" stay in your system. Replace it with "feeling good" until it becomes you!

FEELING GOOD IS YOUR GOAL IN LIFE!

Dance through it!

Change the story!

Change the way you breathe!

Change the puzzle!

Be aware of your forms!

Change them!

You've become a Parkinson's warrior!

Thought for Your Life

Believe in your commitment, visualize it, dream it, expect it, and bring more and more of what you want into your life.

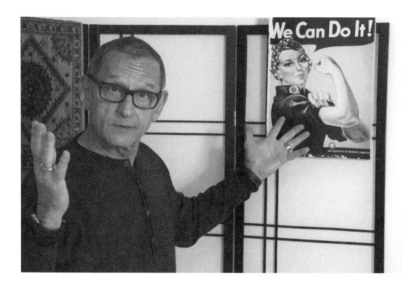

SECTION 4

ADDITIONAL READING

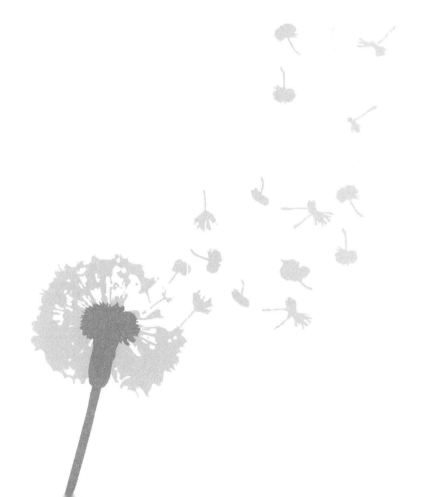

Appendix – The Science

OUR NEURAL NETWORKS

AUTONOMIC NERVOUS SYSTEM

SYMPATHETIC AND PARASYMPATHETIC

VOLTAGE, SPEED, AND RHYTHM

THE BRAIN

THE TRIO

Our Neural Networks

Our brain is able to coordinate our movements, control our bodily functions like breathing, and enable us to feel emotions and sensations like pain, sadness, and happiness through the electrical charges in our neural network.

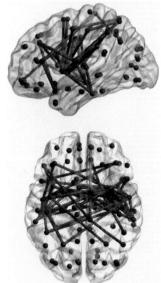

Our brain activity begins with a biochemical stimulus from any of our five senses. When this information reaches our brain, the brain sends its own signal to the body through our spinal cord – the connecting link of our central nervous system.

The brain and body function optimally when each of our neural networks is correctly programmed to produce, send, and receive biochemical information – this free flow of information is the key to our well-being. If there is a biochemical excess, our synapses – the region where nerve impulses are transmitted and received – can get flooded, and the signals can't move on to the next neuron. If there's a deficiency, the nerve signals might have nothing to travel on. As a result, other parts of the body will react to these biochemical excesses or deficiencies by overworking or shutting down. The result could range from anxiety or mental instability to physical illness.

Neurotransmitters are the brain chemicals that communicate information inside our brain and to the rest of our body. The brain uses the neurotransmitters to execute our most important bodily functions – telling our heart to beat, our lungs to breathe, our stomach to digest, and other vital tasks.

When they're out of balance, they can affect virtually every aspect of our being – our mood, sleep, weight, and health. In addition to diet, genetic disposition, drugs, and alcohol, stress and anxiety can cause our neurotransmitters to veer out of balance.

There are two types of neurotransmitters: ones that calm the brain and create balance, and ones that stimulate the brain. When the excitatory neurotransmitters are overactive, they can easily deplete the inhibitory ones to create a chemical imbalance.

Neurotransmitters: Dopamine, Acetylcholine, GABA, and Serotonin

We are going to focus on the four basic neurotransmitters that are specifically related to Parkinson's disease – two excitatory and two inhibitory.

They each have their own function and when they are working properly, they help us arrive at our balanced state of being.

Excitatory

DOPAMINE

Dopamine is our mood guru. It controls our energy and excitement and monitors our metabolism. Associated with the "pleasure system" of our brain, it works like a natural amphetamine to motivate us.

Dopamine has strong ties in the brain to motor coordination, cognition, mood, and attention. The overproduction of dopamine due to hyperstimulation can lead to its depletion over time. This dopamine imbalance can express itself with symptoms like forgetfulness and apathy, or create the environment for the spread of depression, fatigue, and Parkinson's disease.

Dopamine is used up and depleted in our brain-wave state of excitement, especially beta.

ACETYLCHOLINE

This excitatory neurotransmitter lubricates our nervous system to enable more efficient stimulation for cognition, memory, and arousal. It enables energy and information to pass through our internal systems and keeps the signals from dissipating before they reach their destination.

A slower brain speed means a less-rapid reaction time that can lead to reduced cognition, as well as slowed impulses that result in organs functioning less than optimally.

An imbalance of acetylcholine can lead to learning disabilities and memory lapses and is associated with diseases like Alzheimer's and myasthenia gravis.

Inhibitory Neurotransmitters

SEROTONIN

Serotonin is one of the calming neurotransmitters that keep us from entering our survival syndrome. When there's sufficient flow, serotonin provides a sense of satisfaction in our body and mind. We sleep well, feel rested, think rationally, have a good appetite, and enjoy life. We are in our alpha state.

Serotonin is necessary to maintain a stable mood. When dopamine is working overtime at stimulating the brain, there's a danger of serotonin being depleted. An imbalance of serotonin can manifest itself through many conditions, including apathy, obsessive-compulsive disorder, migraines, and anxiety disorders.

GABA

GABA is often called the brain's natural Valium. The chief inhibitory neurotransmitter, it provides us with rhythm and is linked with relaxation and anti-anxiety effects through the production of endorphins and other brain chemicals. A good level of GABA provides a sense of balance between body, mind, and spirit, especially in our rhythm.

When our dopamine is firing too often, GABA is sent out in an attempt to balance the overstimulation. The physical effects of a GABA imbalance could include headaches and hypertension, a sense of anxiety, and dread of being overwhelmed.

How the Neurotransmitters Work Together

Our nervous system works through both biologic stimulation and electric stimulation.

Biologic stimulation comes from dopamine, which opens the nerves, acetylcholine, which oils the nerves and gives them a smooth run, and on the other side, serotonin, which calms the nerves, and GABA, which controls the rhythm.

We're always in a situation of stimulation versus calming. The key is to be in the middle.

When our neurotransmitters – dopamine, serotonin, acetylcholine, and GABA – are balanced, then we're in an alpha state or lower beta state. But if we secrete too much dopamine in a highly anxious state, we can burn out the serotonin that is attempting to counteract it.

If we have too much serotonin, we become apathetic, but if we don't have enough, we may develop anxiety. Where has our middle state home base gone? It's fallen victim to our scripts, the stories we tell ourselves in a perpetual continuum.

Freeze, Fight, Flight

We discussed earlier our ancestors' basics of survival – the three Fs – *freeze, fight, flight*. But we must also realize that to this day, we are employing these instincts all the time.

Freeze

Tremors are not a Parkinson's invention – they are a jungle invention.

When an animal is in a situation before making a decision to fight or run away, it begins to tremble, it changes its body form and the look in its eyes. When it makes that decision to fight or flee, the tremors stop.

Tremors are a genetic freezing condition in everyone – some people get them when they enter the classroom for a big exam, others get it right before they go onstage to perform. We even have a term for it: *stage fright*. Once the test begins or the show starts, the trembling disappears.

Tremors are a freezing genetic jungle behavior pattern – they are movements that are being choked off. In Parkinson's, freezing is the great neutralizer

– someone with Parkinson's is so frozen, they don't do anything, they're unable to either fight or flee.

If a person understands that freezing equals indecision, then it opens the way to do something about it – fight or flight.

Fight

To stop the trembling accompanying stage fright or heading into the big exam, we can either fight our way through and meet the challenge head on, or we can flee, escape the situation, and back down from the challenge. Either way, the tremors stop.

The problem is that the human brain tends to take everything to the extreme. It's not good enough to go onstage and perform well; we suddenly want to be the best, we need to be the best. And even being the best isn't good enough.

By fighting to the extreme – whether it's obsessing about the promotion at work or getting the biggest car on the block – we make ourselves sick, we make our bodies sick. Fight is effective and positive only as long as the body and mind understand they have a common goal to achieve something, and not because of an obsession to be the best or achieve the most.

Anything done to the extreme will exact a grave price. Look at marathon runners or extreme fighters – they do much more damage than good. Don't take it to the extreme!

Flight

Flight is actually a way to subconsciously wipe out things we don't want to deal with. In the modern world, that can mean replacing the challenges we should be facing with obsessive shopping or compulsive eating.

Our flight has become an escape — occurring because we're not aware of our body language and we're unable to translate what our body is saying through our human mind. We have become professional escape artists.

When we're in a freezing situation and we're a professional escape artist, then we flee. We escape from a freezing situation that we don't know how to cope with — it's our basic jungle survival formula.

Where Are We?

It's important for us to be able to recognize if we're in one of the extremes of flight, flight, or freezing. We are always making decisions about whether to fight or escape, and the best situation we can be in is a midstage combination of the three Fs.

Parkinson's sufferers know freezing in the extreme. But freezing can also be a great interval. In the middle of an argument that's getting heated, we can say, "Hey, let's cool out and think about this." Before choosing fight or flight, freezing can be a positive place.

But when we're unable to ever fight or flee, then we become professional freezers. Many of my clients suffer from freezing attacks of upward of two or three hours – but something changes when they begin to understand that they've actually been freezing since they were children.

I hear stories like "My parents never hugged me, they never let me show feelings or fear." They were frozen, feeling-wise!

Feelings = body language! With this realization, I've seen stages of freezing by some clients reduced from three hours to 20 minutes.

They understood that they acquired the habit of freezing under certain situations years ago. And once they received the "legitimacy" of Parkinson's, the freezing got worse – until they decided to do something about it.

Autonomic Nervous System (ANS)

Our autonomic nervous system controls our body systems and automatic bodily functions – but it's also in charge of our survival mode.

It is responsible for the physical responses felt in a phobic reaction. What happens when we're in survival mode?

- Eyes: pupils dilate
- Heart: beats faster and more forcefully
- Lungs: hyperventilation

- Stomach: reduces output of digestive enzymes, producing nausea
- Bowel: movement of food slows down
- Bladder: sphincter muscle constricts
- Blood vessels: main vessels dilate; blood pressure rises.

We are usually unaware of our autonomic nervous system, because it functions involuntarily and reflexively. The ANS regulates the functioning of our internal organs – our heart, stomach, intestines – by controlling the muscles in those organs.

When our heart starts to beat faster or our blood pressure skyrockets, it's the ANS at work.

Our ANS comes into play when we are acting out our scenarios from our alpha state of peace and balance that bring us to our survival syndrome emergency mode.

Sympathetic and Parasympathetic Nervous Systems

The ANS is divided into the sympathetic nervous system and the parasympathetic nervous system.

The sympathetic nervous system stimulates and stores our survival syndrome, and the parasympathetic calms us down. When the sympathetic and the parasympathetic are balanced, we are in our midway – our alpha state.

The sympathetic nervous system takes over when we are stimulated or hyperstimulated and our survival syndrome is triggered: our blood pressure rises, our heart beats faster, digestion slows. Our dopamine and acetylcholine neurotransmitters begin to work overtime.

When we're relaxed and at peace, our parasympathetic nervous system is at work conserving our energy. Our blood pressure can decrease, the pulse rate lessens, and the digestion process is at full power. Our GABA and serotonin are balanced.

Our ideal state is a balance between the parasympathetic and the sympathetic nervous systems. When we're imbalanced toward the sympathetic, we move to our survival syndrome, and when we're imbalanced toward low parasympathetic, we become apathetic and enter a state of freezing.

Where are we at our best? In the middle, of course.

Everything – our heartbeat, breathing, and rhythm – works better in the middle, in a state called *homeostasis*.

The Trio

In order to develop the mind-body relationship, we must understand some basics about how they both work.

As we discussed earlier, we have different types of brain activity. We actually have three brains at work inside of us: the reptilian brain, the mammalian brain, and the Homo sapien – or human – brain. When we are born, we possess only the reptilian and the mammalian brain, which help us deal with the basic elements of survival. We live by the rules of the jungle, focusing only on food, sleep, and survival. For example, place a finger in front of a baby, and he instinctively thinks it's a nipple.

Our mammalian brain is a big advancement over the reptilian, as it possesses the ability to feel and to solve problems of the present. One way we can use to describe our brain is like a computer where we store all of our experiences of the past. Each file on the computer disk tells us how to react to any given situation based on past experiences. It stores all of our instinct and intuition.

"I'm hungry so I will hunt in that place where I got a deer last time." "I'm wet so I will find shelter in the cave by the river."

The reptilian brain doesn't have the feelings and the memory that the mammalian brain does. It lives only according to the survival rules of the jungle – fight, flight, or freeze. It doesn't know how to analyze or to think about the future or the past.

The third member of the trio is the human brain. A baby isn't born with this brain, it only begins to develop with time – gifted with inner dialogue, the ability to analyze situations and to plan for the future based on past experiences and acquired knowledge. The human brain lives in the past, present, and the future and is constantly taking in outside stimuli that is processed, analyzed, and passed on to the body through our nervous system for action.

It's important to remember, however, that our body is equipped with jungle behavior patterns and that this state remains with us throughout our lives! When we are cut off on the road by a reckless driver, we usually don't respond with our human brain, but with our jungle instincts, perhaps impulsively thrusting our middle finger out the window. In that split second, we take our acquired knowledge – everything that's inscribed in our internal computer – and we respond. Only afterward, our human mind starts to work, and we might think, "Did I do the right thing? What could I have done differently?"

This example brings us to a major point we brought up earlier that's worth emphasizing: *the body works much faster than the mind*.

The body feels hunger, fear, anger – and immediately offer solutions before the brain can begin to analyze the situation and provide its own solutions.

Bibliography/Reference Works for Further Reading

Articles

Earhart, PhD, Gammon M. "Dance as Therapy for Individuals with Parkinson's Disease." *European Journal of Physical and Rehabilitation Medicine* 45:2 (June 2009), 231–238. http://www.bu.edu/neurorehab/files/2014/02/Dance-as-Therapy-for-Individuals-with-PD.pdf.

French, Tania Gabrielle. "Why Do Music Conductors Live So Long?" From *The Longevity Guide: Why Do Music Conductors Live into Their 90s?* by Steven Rochlitz, Ph.D. http://www.rethinkingcancer.org/resources/articles/why-do-music-conductors-live-so-long.php.

Mackrell, Judith. "Dance Is Just What the Doctor Ordered." *The Guardian*, November 20, 2014. http://www.theguardian.com/stage/dance-blog/2014/nov/20/dance-for-parkinsons-disease-capturing-grace-therapeutic-benefits.

Books

Campbell, Don. *The Mozart Effect: Tapping the Power of Music to Heal the Body, Strengthen the Mind and Unlock the Creative Spirit*. New York: Quill, 2001.

Carlson, Neil R. *Physiology of Behavior: 11th Edition*. Essex, UK: Pearson, 2012.

Chopra, Deepak. Any book by Deeprak Chopra.

Coleman, Vernon. *Mindpower: How to Use Your Mind to Heal Your Body*. Delhi, India: Indus Publishing, 2005.

Damasio, Antonio. *The Feeling of What Happens: Body and Emotions in the Making of Consciousness*. San Diego, CA: Mariner Books, 2000.

Doidge, Norman. *The Brain That Changes Itself.* Brilliance Audio, 2008.

Haxthausen, Margit and Leman, Rhea. *Body Sense: Exercise for Relaxation*. New York: Pantheon, 1987.

Heller, Joseph and William Henkin. *Bodywise: An Introduction to Hellerwork for Regaining Flexibility and Well-Being*. Berkeley, CA: North Atlantic Books, 2004.

Siever, Larry J. and William Frucht. *New View of Self: How Genes and Neurotransmitters Shape Your Mind, Your Personality, and Your Mental Health*. New York: Macmillan USA, 1997.

Tolle, Eckart. *The Power of Now: A Guide to Spiritual Enlightenment*. Novato, CA: New World Library, 2004.

IMAGES

Diaphragm illustration courtesy of Theresa Knott/en.wikipedia

Caveman fight flight illustration courtesy of Theresa Knott/
en.wikipedia

Alpha beta illustration courtesy of Andreus/Dreamstime.com

Neural network illustration courtesy of http://www.plosone.org/
article/info%3Adoi%2F10.1371%2Fjournal.pone.0057831
© 2013 Hong et al.

Director's clapperboard illustration courtesy of Creative Commons

Academy Award photo courtesy of Creative Commons

Mobile devices photo courtesy of Redjar/Creative Commons

LYRICS

"Feeling Good," by Leslie Bricusse, Anthony Newley, T.R.O. INC.

"Free Your Mind," by Denzil Foster, Thomas Derrick Mcelroy,
Sony/ATV Music Publishing LLC, Next Decade Entertainment, Inc.

"More Than a Feeling," by Donald T. Scholz, Sony/ATV Music
Publishing LLC, Next Decade Entertainment, Inc.

"It's My Life," by Martin Gellner, Max Martin, Jon Bon Jovi, Martin Karl
Sandberg, Richard Sambora, Werner Stranka, Sony/ATV Tunes LLC.

A Message from the Publisher

I thank the world for Alex. He saved my life!

Two years ago, I struggled to lift myself out of the taxi, unable to stand straight, I shuffled down the walkway like a little old man. Three hours later, I danced joyously back down that walkway and into the waiting taxi. I turned to Geraldine, my wife. "What was that? What just happened?!" Alex showed me that, for those few hours, my Parkinson's had disappeared. Where did it go?

In that same year, I made three short trips to Israel and under Alex's eagle eye learned the regime described in this book. Having led a rather sedentary life, this was tough going, and a journey that my mind and body resisted. But seeing symptoms drop away was nothing short of a miracle. Today I have eliminated some 60% or more of my Parkinson's symptoms. I am once again back in the world, productive, creative, and enjoying living in this body. Something I never thought would happen. I joyously do the exercises 30 to 60 minutes every day and continue to find new areas to explore.

Alex works intuitively. He probably doesn't think much about how he does what he does, he just does it. Being both a martial artist and an accomplished jazz musician, he is used to responding in the moment. He doesn't think much about how he will defend himself or what he will play. He just responds to the other musicians or whatever presents itself. He works this way with his clients, too, seeing deeply into their posture, their breathing, heartbeat, eyes, and body language.

His work is so important and so valuable to other Parkinson's people that I knew we had to publish a book. Getting a book out of Alex was no mean feat but writer David Brinn did the impossible. He caught lightning in a bottle by observing Alex at work, drawing him out, organizing a lifetime of experience, and capturing the voice and essence of a true master. Reading the book is like being with Alex in his Israeli studio. "Stop thinking! Dance! Let the music be your teacher."

Make no mistake, this is not Thin-Thighs-in-Thirty-Days. If you are still waiting for a silver bullet to cure your Parkinson's, this program is *not* for you. But if you are willing to do your own heavy lifting and watch your life change for the better, you've come to the right place.

There is one reason that people come from all over the world to work with Alex: he gets results. But this is because he has stacked the deck. The people he works with are — in his words — Parkinson's warriors. They are willing to do the work and it is hard work.

It requires a willingness to give up false beliefs that you may have held on to for a lifetime. It requires you to start listening to your body and get out on the dance floor.

There are only two choices with Parkinson's. You can live out the sad story of the future that your doctor told you

("Parkinson's isn't a death sentence, it's a life sentence")
or you can write a new story for yourself and return to a
level of health that will amaze your doctor, your friends,
and yourself.

Alex's life-long experience in jazz, martial arts, and the
military have blended into a practice that anyone can
do, one that will bring about miracles in their life.

We are thrilled and honored to serve Alex and all
Parkinson's people by publishing this book. May your
adventure to a new body begin now!

Michael Wiese
Publisher, Divine Arts

Acknowledgments

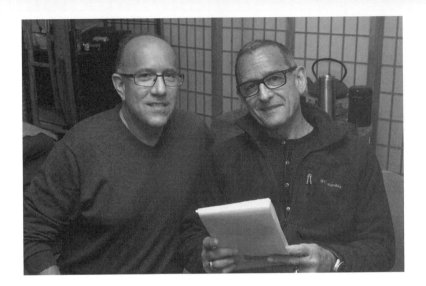

Alex Kerten

I want to thank Alex Kerten (myself) for being where I needed you to be, for the support my mind gave my body and my body gave my mind, and for believing in myself. Thank you.

Thank you to my children – Arik, Shelly, and Anat – and grandchildren – Shani, Sivan, Lihi, Ori, Adi, Amit, and Ido – who accepted me and love me for who I am.

Thank you to my parents who gave me all the freedom I needed to decide what is "good" for me.

A special thank-you to Daniella Har-Paz who assisted me however she could — she's my life partner with one big heart.

Thank you, David Brinn, for helping me to find my writing voice and for the chance to know you for who you are.

Thank you to my brother Emanuel Kerten (Nulli) who has been working with me for a very long time and stood by me for so many years.

Thank you Dorit Nevo and the El-Ron family, who supported me and believed in what I did during our life together.

Thank you to Gad Skolnic, my martial arts master, who gave me so very much in order to get to this day, and who believed in the power that is rooted within us.

Thank you to Michael Wiese and beautiful Geraldine Overton, for believing in my way of life and encouraging the birth of this book.

Thank you to Michal Noy and Shmuel Merhav, real friends who are always willing to give of themselves.

Thank you, Dr. Marieta Anca-Herschkovitsch, Prof. Avner Cohen, Dr. Moshe Kushnir, Dr. Zeev Nitzan, Prof. Rivka Inzelberg, Dr. Rima Schvekher, and Dr. Sharon Hassin for their interest in my work and for their contributions to its advancement.

And, thank you to music, especially jazz, for teaching me what life really is.

I firstly want to thank Alex Kerten, an inspirational colleague and friend who opened up a whole new world to me. His dedication and example have helped make me a better person.

Thanks to Daniella Har-Paz, who made everything run smoothly and enables Alex to dedicate his full attention to his clients.

Thank you to Michael Wiese and Geraldine Overton for putting their faith in me to move onward and upward in spreading this important message.

Thanks to Judy Siegel Itzokovich, Israel's preeminent health and science reporter, for her generous advice and rigorous fact-checking. Thank you, Gary Sunshine, for your amazing editing work and your supernatural attention to detail. A special thank-you to Bonnie Behar Brooks – the matchmaker who had a hunch.

And most of all, thanks to Shelley, my wife of 30 years, and our amazing family – Adina, Yoray, Sarit, Koby, and Matan for their support and love. They are, and will continue to be, my main script for as long as they'll have me.

About the Authors

Alex Kerten, 69, is founder and director of the Gyro-Kinetics Center in Herzliya, Israel. He has been researching anatomy and the physiology of behavior for over 30 years and treats clients with movement disorders, specializing in Parkinson's disease.

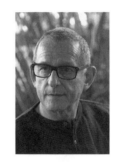

David Brinn, 56, is the managing editor of *The Jerusalem Post*, Israel's leading English newspaper. A native of Portland, Maine, he lives in Ma'aleh Adumim with his wife, Shelley. They have four children. brinnd@gmail.com twitter: davidbjpost

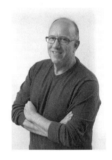

For more info about the book and its authors please see

Website: *www.parkinson-gk.com/english*

Email: *Alex Kerten at: Gyro2014@012.net.il*

Book trailer: *https://youtu.be/mYSqyMkHr4o*

Facebook: *www.facebook.com/GoodbyeParkinsons*

Visit: *Gyro-Kinetics Center, 7 Nehemya St., Hertzliya, Israel*

Testimonials

You can be a healthy person with Parkinson's! It's a very, very important concept that I learned from Alex, and I tell it to my patients all the time.
  – Dr. Marieta Anca-Herschkovitsch, head of the Movement Disorder Clinic, Edith Wolfson Medical Center, Holon, Israel

Alex is doing God's work. Most of the patients he is treating have encountered a problem with a conventional medical establishment that is not always willing to accept changes and innovations. He provides those patients with answers, gives them help, and eases their plight through different means. I think that the bottom line for all of us needs to be "What is good for the patient?" If his treatment works, then it needs to be supported and given exposure.
  – Prof. Avner Cohen, pediatric specialist and director of the Child Center for Clalit Medical Services in Petah Tikva, Israel

Alex Kerten is a pioneer in the field of movement therapy for Parkinson's patients. Only now is the importance of what he does becoming apparent.
  – Dr. Moshe Kushnir, retired Head of Neurology, Kaplan Medical Center, Rehovot, Israel

Alex Kerten has given an answer to Parkinson's conditions for which there are there are no answers in any other kind of treatment. This method is not meant to be instead of conventional treatment but to complement it, and it does that beautifully. But it also gives an answer to aspects of the symptoms that conventional treatment has been unable to.
  He strengthens not only patients' motor skills but also their confidence in themselves. I would recommend anyone with signs of Parkinson's to try Alex's methods.
  – Dr. Zeev Nitzan, neurologist, Barzilai Medical Center, Ashkelon, Israel

What I know about Alex and his Gyro-Kinetics treatment is that it really, really helps my patients. Objectively, I've seen that it gives them energy and the freedom of movement that they've lost. More subjectively, when Parkinson's patients are able to move more freely and regain some of their movements, it does so much for their mental and psychological health and their self-confidence.
  If a qualified medical professional gives an OK that a patient is physically able, I would recommend the Gyro-Kinetics method as a positive supplement to treatment of Parkinson's disease.
  – Prof. Rivka Inzelberg, neurologist specialist and Parkinson's disease specialist at the Tel Aviv University's Sackler Faculty of Medicine and the Sagol Neuroscience Center at Sheba Medical Center, Tel Aviv, Israel

I have many patients who profited from Alex's treatment over the past several years. They have told me that they felt more energetic and alive.
  – Dr. Sharon Hassin, Director, Movement Disorders Institute, Department of Neurology and Sagol Neuroscience Center Chaim Sheba Medical Center, Israel

I've been a psychiatrist for 40 years and have treated countless Parkinson's patients. There's always a difference between patients who are doing something for themselves like keeping active and those who are doing nothing.

When I met Alex and learned about his work, I realized immediately that he was helping his clients. One of my patients went to him and after a week he was a different person. He was happy — even with Parkinson's and his troubles. Alex is able to help people not only physically but also in changing their mental outlook.

– Dr. Rima Schvekher, clinical psychologist, Tel Aviv

Last year, I was running around the mountains near my home like a gazelle. Now, a year after I was diagnosed with Parkinson's, I became so afraid of falling over that I almost stopped taking walks.

A friend suggested that I meet with Alex. We talked about my father, who died 10 years ago. I didn't like him, he wasn't a very nice person. Alex kept telling me that my whole situation was because of my father. I don't want to believe in that shit, but of course, it makes perfect sense.

When we meet, Alex talks a lot and I cry a lot. But I feel so much better after I've been there and cried my eyes out and jumped around with the exercises. When I come back home, my friends say they can see the difference in the way I'm moving. I'm lighter.

I hurt my body for many years — it was shouting out to me, but I just didn't listen. Thanks to Alex, I now listen to it.

– Hella Latthigsen, dairy farmer, Negev, Israel

The most devastating feeling of newly diagnosed Parkinson's patients is helplessness against a chronic disease that seems to offer a dark future. But Alex Kerten — with his experience, imagination, and enthusiasm — has created a method that gives them hope for better coping and even improvement — using exercises and a new way of thinking. With the aging of the population, Parkinson's and other neurological conditions can strike virtually anyone, and his book will come to the rescue for many of them.

– Judy Siegel-Itzkovich, health and science editor, of *The Jerusalem Post*

As Tel Aviv director of the Israel Parkinson's Association, I meet with new members and offer advice. One of the first things I suggest is a visit to Alex, because I've found that he has solutions to 99% of the problems they are encountering.

I've been using the Gyro-Kinetics method for four years, and it gives me so much hope. I arrive there as a sick person, and I leave as a healthy person. It's having Parkinson's but feeling like you don't have Parkinson's.

– Yehudit Raz, director of the Tel Aviv chapter of the Israel Parkinson's Association

ALSO FROM DIVINE ARTS

....

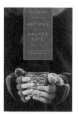

RECIPES FOR A SACRED LIFE:
True Stories and a Few Miracles
Rivvy Neshama   2013 IPPY Gold Award Winner

"Neshama's stories are uplifting, witty, and wise: one can't go wrong with a recipe like that. The timeless wisdom she serves up is food for the soul."
—Publishers Weekly

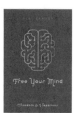

FREE YOUR MIND: *A Meditation Guide to Freedom and Happiness*
Ajay Kapoor

"Free Your Mind goes beyond today's fashionable mindfulness movement by using our thinking, rather than simply noting it. Kapoor carefully shows us how to use our minds to break down our mental conditioning and become truly free."
— Franz Metcalf, author of What Would Buddha Do?

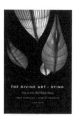

THE DIVINE ART OF DYING: *How to Live Well While Dying*
Karen Speerstra & Herbert Anderson, Foreword by Ira Byock, MD

"A magnificent achievement. The Divine Art of Dying is a moving and inspiring book about taking control of your life as it starts to come to a close."
— Will Schwalbe, author of the New York Times-bestselling The End of Your Life Book Club

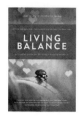

LIVING IN BALANCE: *A Mindful Guide for Thriving in a Complex World*
Joel & Michelle Levey, Foreword by His Holiness the Dalai Lama

"Joel and Michelle have constructed a text of sheer brilliance. Every page offers new insights and truth."
—Caroline M. Myss, PhD, author of Why People Don't Heal and How They Can and Anatomy of the Spirit

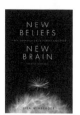

NEW BELIEFS, NEW BRAIN: *Free Yourself from Stress and Fear*
Lisa Wimberger

"Lisa has captured an ageless wisdom and has rephrased it in modern parlance, bringing a new level of approachability to the teachings of our spiritual forebears."
— Dr. David Perlmutter, author of Power Up Your Brain: The Neuroscience of Enlightenment

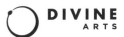

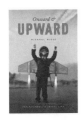

ONWARD & UPWARD: *Reflections of a Joyful Life*
Michael Wiese   2014 COVR Award Winner

"Onward & Upward is the memoir of a rare and wonderful man who has lived a truly extraordinary life. It's filled with Michael Wiese's adventures, his incredible journeys, and his interactions with amazing people."
—**John Robbins, author of** *Diet for a New America*

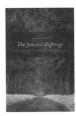

THE JEWELED HIGHWAY: *On the Quest for a Life of Meaning*
Ralph White

"Ralph White's luminous memoirs embrace the spiritual sphere of multiple revelations and portray a love of Gaia, our planet, as perhaps no one has done before. The Jeweled Highway is vital and alive and not constrained by ideology or political correctness. It is Dionysian, a voyage without a plan, a trust in serendipity, an appreciation of love over logic."
—**Thomas Moore, author of** *Care of the Soul*

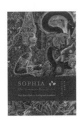

SOPHIA—THE FEMININE FACE OF GOD:
Nine Heart Paths to Healing and Abundance
Karen Speerstra   2013 Nautilus Silver Medalist

"Karen Speerstra shows us most compellingly that when we open our hearts, we discover the wisdom of the Feminie all a round us. A totally refreshing exploration and beautifully researched read."
—**Michael Cecil, author of** *Living at the Heart of Creation*

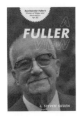

A FULLER VIEW: *Buckminster Fuller's Vision of Hope and Abundance for All*
L. Steven Sieden

Internationally renowned futurist, poet, philosopher, and engineer Dr. R. Buckminster Fuller had a keen awareness that we're all in this life together. For all its genius, his legacy has yet to be fully uncovered — until now.

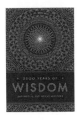

2500 YEARS OF WISDOM:
Sayings of the Great Masters
D.W. Brown

The wisdom from the greatest minds on earth — all in one place.

"The privilege of a lifetime is being who you are."
—**Joseph Campbell**

Celebrating the sacred in everyday life.

Divine Arts was founded to share some of the new and ancient knowledge that is rapidly emerging from the scientific, indigenous, and wisdom cultures of the world, and to present new voices that express eternal truths in innovative, accessible ways.

Although the Earth appears to be in a dark state of affairs, we have realized from the shifts in our own consciousness that millions of beings are seeking and finding a new and optimistic understanding of the nature of reality; and we are committed to sharing their evolving insights.

Our esteemed authors, masters and teachers from around the world, have come together from all spiritual practices to create Divine Arts books. Our unity comes in celebrating the sacredness of life and in having the intention that our work will assist in raising human consciousness and benefiting all sentient beings.

We trust that our work will serve you, and we welcome your feedback.

Michael Wiese, *Publisher*

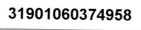